AAOS
American Academy of Orthopaedic Surgeons

ECSI
Emergency Care & Safety Institute

Wilderness First Aid

FIELD GUIDE

THIRD EDITION

Boy Scouts of America

Authors

Alton L. Thygerson, EdD, FAWM

Steven M. Thygerson, PhD, MSPH, CIH

Justin S. Thygerson, PhD, CSP

Medical Editors

Alfonso Mejia, MD, MPH, FAAOS

Bob Elling, MPA, EMT-P

World Headquarters
Jones & Bartlett Learning
25 Mall Road
Burlington, MA 01803
978-443-5000
info@jblearning.com
www.jblearning.com
www.psglearning.com

Jones & Bartlett Learning books and products are available through most bookstores and online booksellers. To contact the Jones & Bartlett Learning Public Safety Group directly, call 800-832-0034, fax 978-443-8000, or visit our website, www.psglearning.com.

American Academy of Orthopaedic Surgeons

Editorial Credits
Chief Commercial Officer: Anna Salt Troise, MBA
Director, Publishing: Hans J. Koelsch, PhD
Senior Manager, Editorial: Lisa Claxton Moore
Senior Editor: Steven Kellert

Bomber planes carried a team of about six airmen. A pilot flew the plane while a navigator followed the route and operated the radio. Others dropped the bombs and fired machine guns at enemy aircraft.

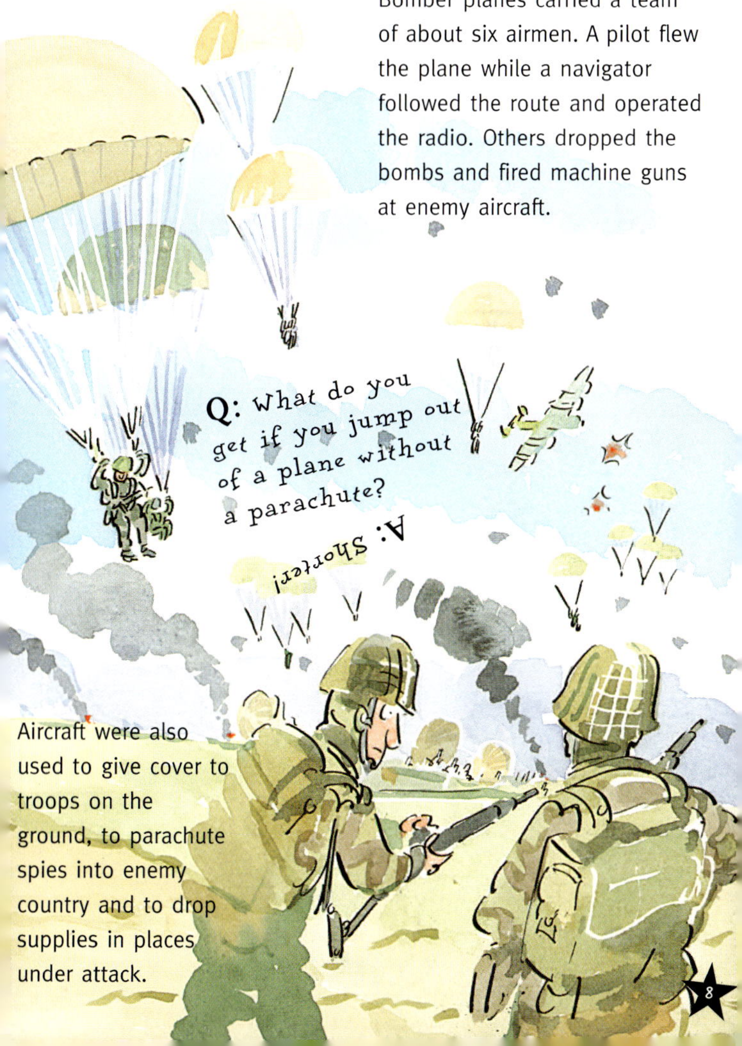

Q: What do you get if you jump out of a plane without a parachute?

A: Shorter!

Aircraft were also used to give cover to troops on the ground, to parachute spies into enemy country and to drop supplies in places under attack.

Secrets and spies

During the war both sides employed spies to find out what the enemy was planning. If spies were captured they were usually tortured or shot.

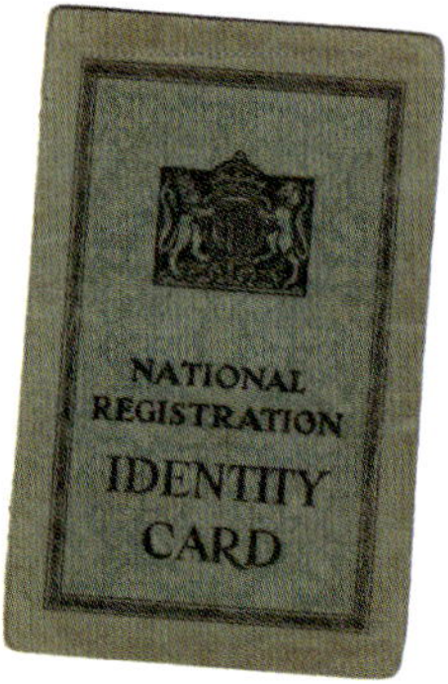

Adults carried identity cards to prove they weren't German spies!

In Britain, many spies worked for the Special Operations Executive (SOE). They operated in enemy territory carrying simple equipment for spying, armed only with a revolver and a knife.

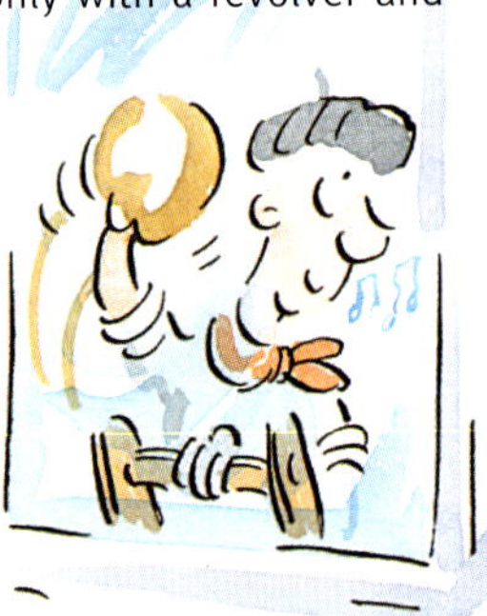

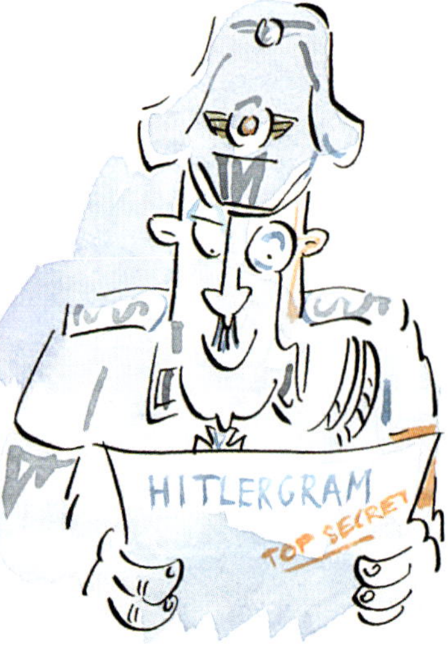

Q: What do you call a spy when he goes to bed?

A: An undercover agent!

Both sides in the war used codes to send secret messages. At Bletchley Park, near Milton Keynes, mathematicians developed an early type of computer to decipher German codes. Valuable information then fell into Britain's hands.

Lookout!

Look out for code-breaking machines at Bletchley Park. Find out what you score on page 14.

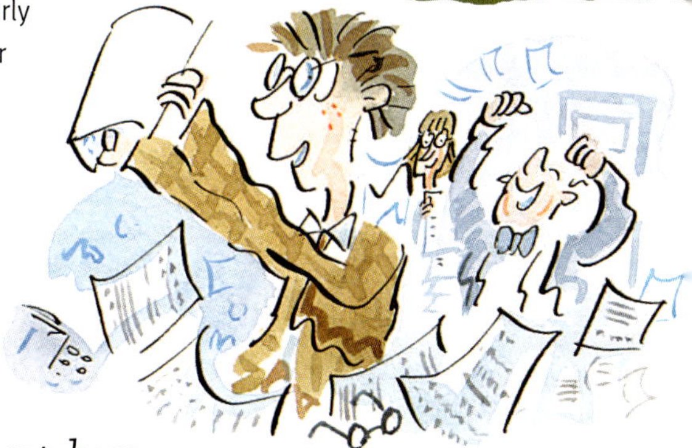

When you get home ...

... decipher this code! Unjumble the words to find out the name of the famous code machine used by Germans to send messages. The code was deciphered at Bletchley Park. It was an exceptionally difficult task because the codes changed every day!

TEH _ _ _

GNIAEM _ _ _ _ _ _

CEDO _ _ _ _

MAIHNCE _ _ _ _ _ _ _

Answer: The Enigma Code Machine

Women in uniform

Women could choose to join the armed forces such as the Women's Auxiliary Air Force (WAAF), the Women's Royal Naval Service (WRNS) and the Auxiliary Territorial Service (ATS). But they were not allowed to fight.

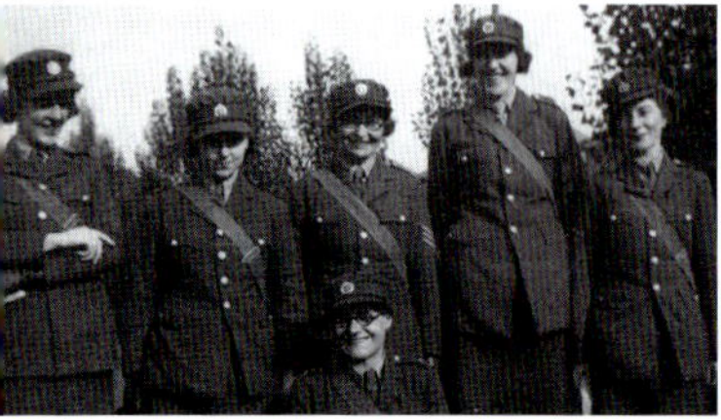

These women belonged to the ATS.

Women in the ATS became army nurses, drove trucks and kept watch for enemy attacks.

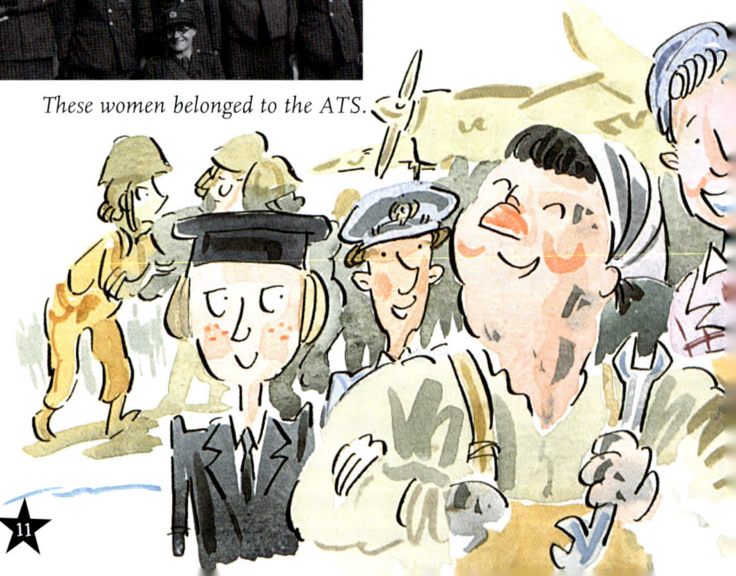

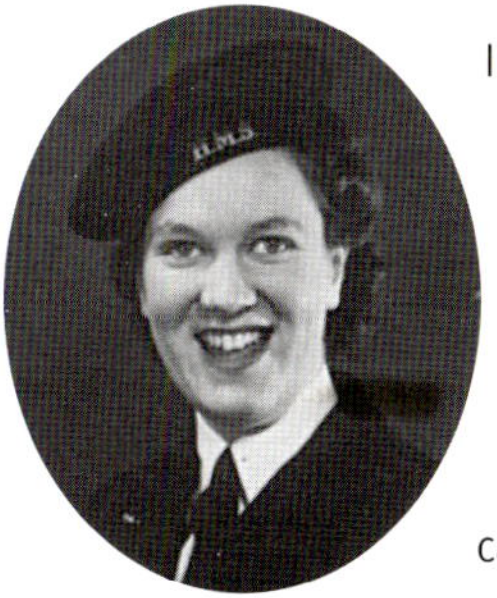

In the WRNS, or Wrens as they were known, women repaired ships and weapons and plotted the routes of enemy and friendly ships. In the WAAF, women mapped the positions of friendly and enemy aircraft, operated radios and manned canteens on airbases.

This Wren worked in payment offices.

Lookout!

Look out for women's uniforms in museum displays about WWII. Find out what you score on page 14.

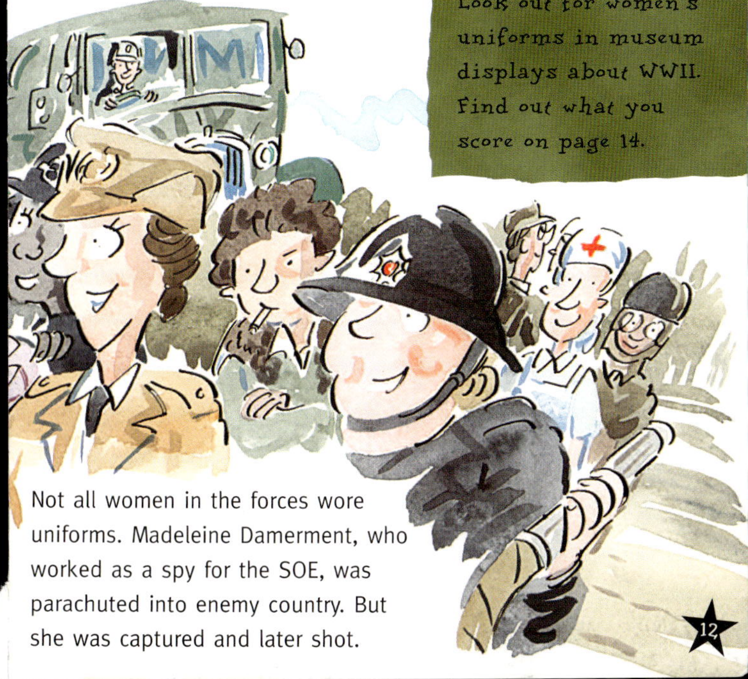

Not all women in the forces wore uniforms. Madeleine Damerment, who worked as a spy for the SOE, was parachuted into enemy country. But she was captured and later shot.

How to use the stickers

First find what you've got to look for under **Lookout!**
Then peel off a sticker with the right number of points and stick it in the blank circle.

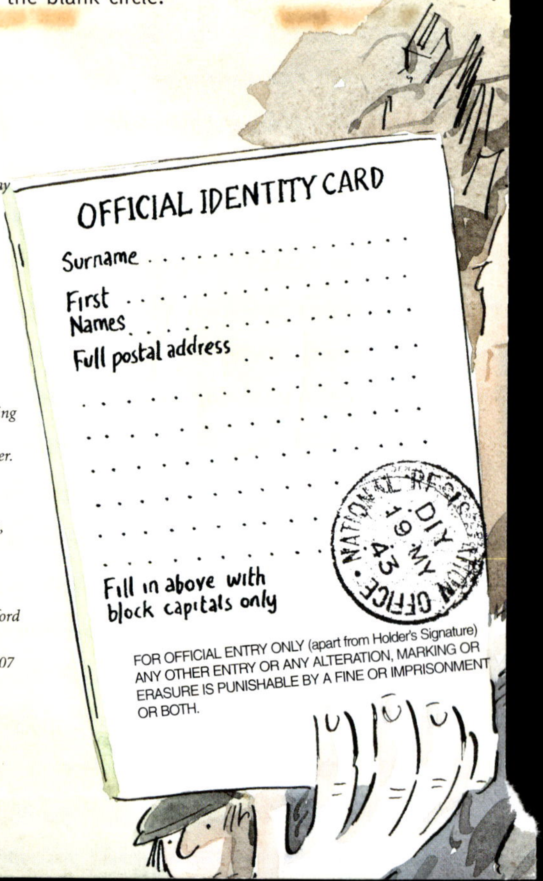

Text: Elizabeth Newbery.

Design: Linda Francis.

Main illustrations: © Clinton Banbury.

Images © and by kind permission: p4 Pitkin Publishing Ltd; p2, 6, 9, 11 and 12 Miss B Pillow; p7 Mr D Stocker.

Production: N&E.

Publication in this form © Pitkin Publishing Ltd, 2003, latest reprint 2007.

Concept & text: © N&E 2003, 3 North St, Osney Island, Oxford OX2 0AY.

ISBN 978-1-84165-118-7 3/07

This textbook is intended solely as a guide to the appropriate procedures to be employed when rendering emergency care to the sick and injured. It is not intended as a statement of the standards of care required in any particular situation, because circumstances and the patient's physical condition can vary widely from one emergency to another. Nor is it intended that this textbook shall in any way advise emergency personnel concerning legal authority to perform the activities or procedures discussed. Such local determination should be made only with the aid of legal counsel.

25481-5

Production Credits

Vice President, Product Management: Marisa R. Urbano
Vice President, Product Operations: Christine Emerton
Director, Product Management: Laura Carney
Director, Content Management: Donna Gridley
Manager, Content Strategy: Tiffany Sliter
Content Strategist: Ashley Procum
Manager, Project Management: Kristen Rogers
Project Manager: John Fuller
Director of Marketing Operations: Brian Rooney
Content Services Manager: Colleen Lamy
VP, Manufacturing and Inventory Control: Therese Connell
Project Management: S4Carlisle Publishing Services
Composition: S4Carlisle Publishing Services
Cover and Text Design: Scott Moden
Senior Media Development Editor: Troy Liston
Rights & Permissions Manager: John Rusk
Rights Specialist: Liz Kincaid
Cover and title page images: © Bruce Port/Moment/Getty Images.
Printing and Binding: Vintage Graphic Solutions, Inc

Library of Congress Cataloging-in-Publication Data

Names: Thygerson, Alton L., author. | Thygerson, Steven M., author. | Thygerson, Justin S., author. | American Academy of Orthopaedic Surgeons, author.
Title: Wilderness first aid field guide / Alton Thygerson, Steve Thygerson, Justin Thygerson, AAOS.
Description: Third edition. | Burlington : Jones & Bartlett Learning, [2023]
Identifiers: LCCN 2021055037 | ISBN 9781284254815 (spiral bound)
Subjects: LCSH: Mountaineering injuries. | Outdoor medical emergencies. | First aid in illness and injury.
Classification: LCC RC88.9 .M6 T49 2023 | DDC 617.1/0276522--dc23/eng/20211201
LC record available at https://lccn.loc.gov/2021055037

6048

Printed in the United States of America
28 27 26 25 10 9 8 7 6 5

Contents

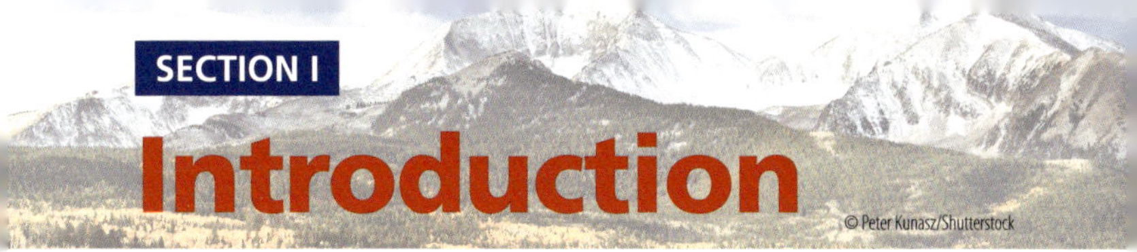

SECTION I

Introduction

Wilderness First Aid

Everyone should be prepared for injuries and medical problems when in situations (eg, the wilderness) in which professional medical care is not readily available. The Wilderness Medical Society defines *wilderness* as a remote geographic location being more than 1 hour from definitive medical care **FIGURE 1**. Thus, you may be in a wilderness environment without realizing it. Some activities, places, and events that can cause you to be in a wilderness situation include the following:

- Recreation (eg, campers, hikers, hunters, rafters, birders, skiers, and climbers)
- Occupations (eg, farmers, foresters, ranchers, and state and national park rangers)
- Remote residences (eg, small communities, farms, ranches, and off-the-grid homes)
- Developing countries
- Urban areas with overwhelmed emergency medical services (EMS) after a natural or human-caused disaster

Those far from medical help may be confronted with the following:

- Delayed or prolonged evacuation because of bad weather, a difficult location, or a lack of transportation or communication

- Adverse conditions (eg, heat, cold, rain, snow, and altitude)
- Limited first aid supplies and equipment (eg, restricted to portable and/or improvisation)
- Injuries and illnesses not typically seen in urban areas (eg, altitude illness, frostbite, and wild animal attacks)
- The need for advanced care (eg, reducing some dislocations and wound care)
- The need to make difficult decisions (eg, CPR and evacuation)

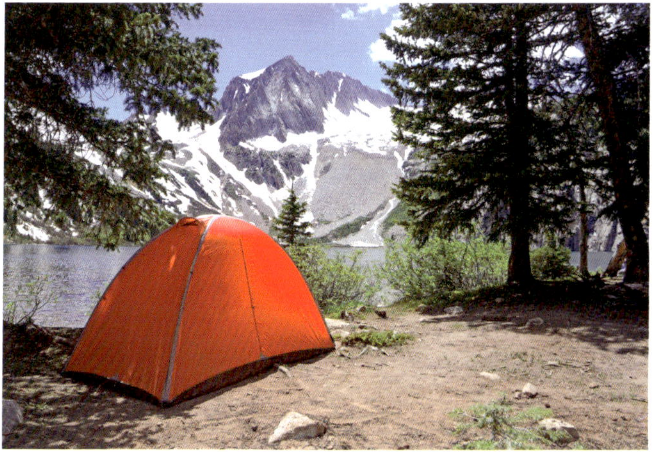

FIGURE 1 Wilderness is defined as any remote geographic location more than 1 hour from definitive professional medical care.

The purpose of this guide is to prepare you to assess and provide care in the above situations. It contains current emergency care recommendations from the Wilderness Medical Society's *Practice Guidelines for Wilderness Emergency Care* and the American Academy of Orthopaedic Surgeons' book *Wilderness First Aid: Emergency Care in Remote Locations,* protocols from the National Association of EMS Physicians and the State of Alaska Cold Injuries Guidelines, the International Liaison Committee on Resuscitation (ILCOR) guidelines, and current medical literature.

These guidelines should not be considered final, as they will be constantly updated to reflect current standards of care. The authors and publisher will not be held responsible, nor assume liability, in respect to the accuracy or implementation of the information or treatment guidelines in this guide.

Abbreviations/Mnemonics Used

AVPU = alert and aware, responds to voice, responds to pain, unresponsive

CPR = cardiopulmonary resuscitation

DOTS = deformity, open wounds, tenderness, swelling

SAMPLE = symptoms, which are the subjective physical and mental features of an illness or injury as described by the person, including the chief complaint; allergies; medications; pertinent past history; last food/fluids; and events leading up to the illness or injury

RICE = rest, ice, compression, elevation

ASAP = as soon as possible

Finding Out What Is Wrong: Assessment

A good assessment is essential to finding the problem to be treated and determining if first aid or professional medical care is needed. The saying, "find it; fix it," stresses that you cannot provide first aid unless you know what is wrong.

Check a person systematically. Do this by performing these four steps:

1. Scene Size-Up
2. Primary Assessment
3. Secondary Assessment with three parts:
   - **A.** Physical Exam
   - **B.** SAMPLE History
   - **C.** Optional assessments (vital signs)
4. Documentation

In most cases:

1. Take charge of the situation. You should have already made a decision about helping those in need of first aid. Identify yourself as a first aid provider to the person and bystanders. If someone is already in charge, ask whether you can help.
2. Obtain permission (known as consent) from the person to help. Consent is implied for an unresponsive person, a responsive person who remains silent and does not resist receiving first aid, and for children when a parent is not available.
3. Protect yourself from contact with blood and/or other body fluids by wearing disposable gloves and glasses, when available.

A barrier device is recommended when giving breaths during CPR. If possible, wash your hands with soap and water, rubbing hands and fingers for at least 20 seconds, before providing care, and definitely wash your hands after giving first aid.

4. Most people do not require a complete assessment (described below).
5. If you find a significant medical problem during an assessment, stop and immediately provide treatment.
6. Emergencies may require attracting the attention of rescuers. Yell for help or use a whistle to attract nearby bystanders. You may have to send another person(s) for help. Other means of seeking help include using a phone or a radio. Using the techniques found in the *Signaling for Help* section of this field guide can attract rescuers.

1. Scene Size-Up

As you approach the scene, ask yourself these questions:

A. **Is it safe for you, the injured or ill person(s), and any by-stander(s)?** If the scene appears dangerous, stay away and seek help from trained rescuers. **DO NOT** try a rescue that you have not been trained for. You cannot help the person if you also become injured or ill.

B. **How many people are involved?** There could be more than one person, so look around and ask about others. If there are two or more injured or ill people, go to the quiet, motionless person(s) first.

C. **What is wrong?** Form a first impression of the person by asking yourself if they are: (1) injured or ill, (2) responsive or unresponsive, (3) breathing normally, and/or (4) bleeding severely.

D. **How was the person injured or how did they become ill?** Look for clues about what caused the injury or the nature of the illness.

2. Primary Assessment

The purpose of the primary assessment is to identify and treat life-threatening problems requiring immediate care. If you find a life-threatening problem, stop and treat it before continuing through the assessment. Injured or ill people fall into one of two types: unresponsive or responsive.

For an Alert, Responsive Person: RAP-ABC-DE

You are more likely to see this type of person. Use **RAP-ABC-DE** to recall the sequence of what to do.

R – Check **responsiveness** by making eye contact, introducing yourself, and asking if you can help. The person may give permission for you to help by saying yes or nodding their head.

A – **Ask** the person, "What happened?" and "Where do you hurt?" (known as the chief complaint). If the person appears to be severely injured or ill, **ask** another person(s) to go or to call for help by using a mobile phone, satellite phone, or radio.

P – **Position** the person in a comfortable position (such as lying down or leaning against a stable object).

A – Maintain open **airway**. A person who can talk has an open airway.

B – Monitor **breathing**—are there abnormal breathing sounds (such as wheezing, gurgling, snoring)? This field guide covers breathing problems in several other sections.

C – Check **circulation**—is there severe bleeding (blood spurting or rapidly flowing from a wound)? For how to control bleeding, refer to the *Bleeding and Wound Care* section of this field guide.

Continue the assessment. See the following section for completing the **D** and **E** parts of the assessment.

D – **Disability.** Tell the alert person not to move. Whenever you suspect a head or spinal injury, have a bystander stabilize the person's head by holding it still. A more decisive check for spinal injuries happens later during the Physical Exam, while checking the arms and legs. Refer to the *Head Injuries* and *Spinal Cord Injury* sections in this field guide.

E – **Environment** and **Exposure.** Prolonged exposure to extreme temperatures (cold and heat) can threaten life. Such conditions may point to the cause of the person's problem.

Clothing may have to be removed down to the skin to check and treat an injury. If you need to remove clothing, explain what you intend to do and why to the person and bystanders. Remove only as much clothing as necessary, try to maintain privacy, and prevent exposure to cold. Once an injury has been treated, it is important to cover it back up when possible.

For a Motionless, Unresponsive Person: RAB-CAB-DE

These steps resemble the same steps for starting cardiopulmonary resuscitation (CPR)—**RAB-CAB-DE**—although most unresponsive persons do not need CPR.

R – Check **responsiveness** by tapping the person's shoulder and shouting "Are you OK?"

A – If there is no response, **activate** EMS by asking another person(s) to go or call for help by using a mobile phone, satellite phone, or radio.

B – **Breathing?** With the person face up on a flat, firm surface, observe the person's torso between the neck and waist for movement (rise and fall); take 5–10 seconds. If the person is breathing and no spinal injury is suspected, place them on their side and check for severe bleeding.

C – If the person is not breathing or only gasping, give CPR starting with 30 **chest compressions**—push hard; push fast. Use the same beat as the Bee Gee's song, "Stayin' Alive."

A – Open the **airway** by tilting the head back and lifting the chin to move the tongue away from the back of the throat. Do this for all persons, even when spinal injury is suspected.

B – Give two **breaths** (each lasting 1 second and making the chest rise).

Continue cycles of 30 compressions and 2 rescue breaths until an AED arrives, another trained person takes over, you are too exhausted to continue, the scene becomes unsafe, or the person revives. If you do not know CPR, give continuous chest compressions without breaths.

For an unresponsive, normal-breathing person, maintain an open airway, monitor breathing, and continue the assessment.

3. Secondary Assessment

This assessment consists of three parts: Physical Exam, Vital Signs, and SAMPLE History.

A. Physical Exam

First aid providers will find it difficult to avoid close contact with an injured or sick person. However, during a physical exam, first aid providers should wear personal protective equipment and, whenever possible, minimize touching or feeling the person they are helping.

To avoid touching or feeling a person, the physical exam uses these instructions: ***look for*** and ***ask about*** **DOTS**. Three of these four conditions can be accomplished by looking, while the fourth, tenderness, involves asking about and/or having the person who you are helping press or feel a body area for pain or tenderness (if they are capable). The person may tell you about tender or painful areas but it is still important to have them feel for tender areas because the brain generally only focuses on one pain source at a time. During the physical exam head-to-toe check, the first aid provider checks one part of the body at a time by ***looking for*** and ***asking about*** **DOTS**.

Most people require only a physical exam of the body area localized by the chief complaint; a full body physical exam (described below) is not needed. Just as in the Primary Assessment, any life-threatening injuries should be immediately treated before continuing through an assessment. Otherwise, complete the entire Secondary Assessment before treating an injury.

Check a part of the body by ***looking for*** and ***asking about*** **DOTS**:

D: Deformity—abnormal shape of the body part (compare it against the opposite uninjured part). Deformities occur when bones are broken or joints are dislocated.

O: Open wounds—the skin is broken and bleeding is seen.

T: Tenderness—have the person feel their body part and report any tenderness, pain, aches, and where they hurt.

S: Swelling—area looks larger than usual. This is caused by excess fluid in the tissue. Compare one side of the body with the other side (eg, if an ankle appears swollen, compare it with the uninjured ankle).

For a responsive and alert person:

Before starting the physical exam, tell the person what you are going to do. Start at the head and examine each body area by looking for and asking about DOTS.

Check the body areas in the following sequence, starting at the head and checking arms and hands last:

- Head and neck
- Eyes, ears, nose, and mouth
- Shoulders
- Chest and abdomen
- Hips
- Legs and feet
- Arms and hands

If a back, buttocks, or spinal injury is suspected, use others to help roll the person onto their side, keeping the person's nose and navel pointing in the same direction. **DO NOT** twist the torso or neck. Check for DOTS.

Medical Identification Tag

A person with a medical problem or problems may be wearing a medical identification tag (such as on a bracelet or necklace) containing the wearer's medical problem(s) and a 24-hour telephone number. The tag can sometimes help identify what may be wrong with the person. If looking in a wallet or a purse (note: this might be illegal in some states) for medical identification, always have another person present to avoid later accusations should money or credit cards be missing.

B. SAMPLE History

A SAMPLE history helps identify what is wrong. Often the person can tell you, but if they cannot, the information may be obtained from family, friends, bystanders, or a medical identification tag.

S = Symptoms	"What is wrong? Where do you hurt?" (known as the primary complaint or chief complaint)
A = Allergies	"Are you allergic to anything?"
M = Medications	"Are you taking any medications? What are they for? When were they last taken?"
P = Pertinent medical history	"Have you had this problem before? Do you have other medical problems?"
L = Last food/fluids	"When did you last eat or drink anything? What was it? How much? When was the last time you urinated or defecated? Were they normal?"
E = Events leading up to the injury or illness	Injury: "How did you get hurt?" Illness: "What led to this problem?"

For a chief complaint involving an illness, you cannot diagnose the exact cause of the illness. Instead, determine if it is serious enough to require professional medical care.

C. Optional Assessments: Vital Signs

First aid providers are not usually expected to take vital signs (eg, heart rate, breathing rate). Vital signs can show a person's overall condition rather than a specific problem. They show what is going on inside the body. Taking vital signs at 15-minute intervals over time can indicate whether the person is getting better, getting worse, or remaining about the same. The vital signs include: level of responsiveness, heart rate, breathing rate, and skin condition.

Level of Responsiveness: AVPU Scale

A person's level of responsiveness can range from fully responsive (conscious) to unresponsive (unconscious). The four-level AVPU scale describes the person's responsiveness. The scale indicates how the brain is doing.

AVPU Scale

A	**Alert** and aware (eyes open; can answer questions clearly; knows name, where they are, and day of the week)
V	Responds to **Voice** in some way when spoken to (attempts to speak, groans, or moves)
P	Responds to **Pain** (responds to pinching of skin next to the neck above the collarbone—when pinching, **DO NOT** injure the person)
U	**Unresponsive** (no response to Voice or Pain)

Heart Rate (HR)

The heart rate (also known as the pulse rate) is the number of heartbeats per minute. The normal rate for an adult at rest is between 60 and 100 beats per minute. An exception is an athlete in good health with a normal resting heart rate between 40 and 50 beats per minute. Be concerned about the adult whose heart rate stays above 100 or below 60 beats per minute. If the heart rate is taken several times and the person maintains it above 120 beats or below 50 beats per minute, something may be seriously wrong that requires professional medical care.

Measure the heart rate by placing the flat part of the ends of your index and middle fingers 2 inches above the base of the thumb on the inside of the wrist (known as the radial pulse site). **DO NOT** use your thumb, because you might feel your own pulse. Count the beats for 30 seconds, then multiply by 2 to get the heart rate in beats per minute.

A heartbeat felt at the wrist (radial pulse) indicates that enough blood pressure exists to saturate all the body tissues with oxygenated blood.

Breathing Rate (BR)

One breath consists of one inhalation and one exhalation. The breathing rate (also known as the respiration rate) is the number of breaths taken in one minute. The normal breathing rate of an adult at rest is 12 to 20 breaths per minute. A rate less than 8 or greater than 24 is abnormal and may indicate a problem requiring supplemental oxygen.

Count the breathing rate by watching the person's torso between the neck and waist rise and fall for 30 seconds, counting each time the person inhales and then multiplying this number by 2. Some people may deliberately change their breathing rate if they know you are counting them. Try to count the breathing without the person's knowledge by pretending to be taking the heart rate.

Abnormal sounds such as gurgling, crowing, wheezing, snoring, or gasping can indicate a medical problem.

Skin Condition: Color, Temperature, and Moisture

Skin color, especially in light-skinned people, reflects the circulation under the skin as well as oxygen status. For those with dark complexions, changes might not be readily apparent but can be assessed in all people by the appearance of the nail beds, the inside of the lips, and/or under the eyelids.

Get a rough idea of skin temperature by putting the inside of your wrist or the back of your hand on the person's forehead to determine whether the temperature is elevated or decreased. If unsure, try comparing the person's temperature with a known healthy person. Dry skin is normal. Skin that is wet, moist (unless the person has been sweating or in water), or excessively dry and hot suggests a problem.

4. Documentation

For medical and legal reasons, a report should be written as soon as possible, but this should not interfere with a person's treatment. The following SOAP method enables you to document the incident quickly and accurately. Without detracting from the treatment, taking photos as soon as possible of the scene and the injury may be helpful for legal reasons or later professional medical care.

SOAP method:

S = Subjective	What were you told in the SAMPLE history?
O = Objective	What did you find during the scene size-up, primary assessment, and physical exam?
A = Assessment	What do you think was wrong?
P = Plan	What are you going to do for each problem? Is professional medical care needed? Should the person be evacuated?

SOAP Note (example)

Person's Name:________________________________
Date & Time of Incident:__________________________
Age:_____ Gender:______ Location:_______________
Weather:________________

S – Subjective: What did the person tell you? (based upon SAMPLE history)

S = Symptoms/chief complaint(s):	1.
	2.
	3.
A = Allergies:	
M = Medications:	
P = Pertinent medical history:	
L = Last food/fluids:	
E = Events leading up to the injury/illness:	

O – Objective: What did you observe?

Physical exam (includes DOTS)

Head:	Abdomen:
Neck:	Hips:
Eyes, ears, nose, mouth:	Legs, feet, back, buttocks:
Shoulders:	Arms and hands:
Chest:	Medical ID tag:

A – Assessment: What do you think is wrong?

1.	3.
2.	4.

P – Plan: What are you going to do for each of the problems in the Assessment section?

First aid given for each problem	Medical care needed? Yes or No	Evacuate? If yes, how?
1.		
2.		
3.		
4.		

Verbal First Aid: What to Say to a Person

Avoid negative statements that may add to person's distress, fear, and pain. Use simple words to create confidence, comfort, and cooperation.

1. Your first words to a person are very important.
2. **DO NOT** ask unnecessary questions (eg, "What did you do?") unless it aids treatment or satisfies the person's need to talk.
3. Make no judgments.
4. Link a suggestion that you want the injured person to accept with a statement they cannot deny (eg, "That leg is probably hurting, but we'll soon make you comfortable").
5. Tears and/or laughter can be normal—tell the injured person this if such responses seem to make them feel embarrassed or guilty.
6. Stress the positive, but be realistic (eg, instead of "You will not have any pain," say "You will feel better").
7. **DO NOT** deny the obvious (eg, instead of saying, "There is nothing wrong," say, "You've had quite a fall and probably don't feel too good, but we're going to look after you"). **DO NOT** make any promises that you cannot keep (eg, saying "Everything will be OK").

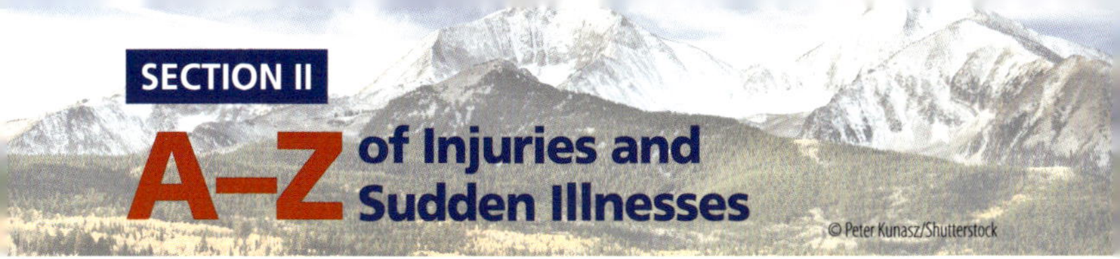

SECTION II

A–Z of Injuries and Sudden Illnesses

© Peter Kunasz/Shutterstock

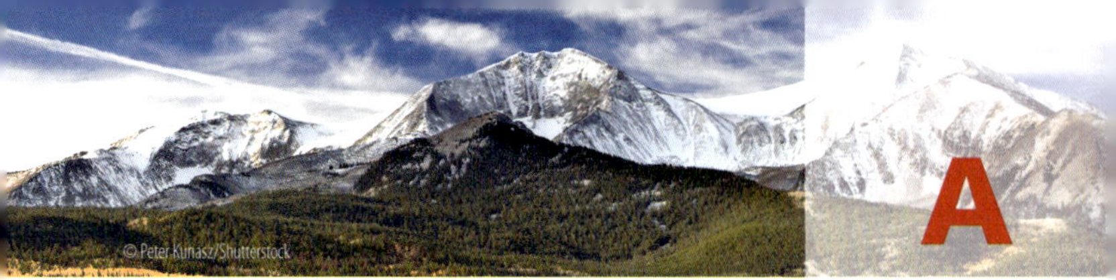

© Peter Kunasz/Shutterstock

Abdominal Complaints

Abdominal Pain

There are many possible causes of abdominal pain, some not so serious and some life threatening. Some can be serious enough to require immediate evacuation for medical care. Illnesses affecting the abdomen have two things in common: they are very painful, and even skilled physicians may have trouble pinpointing an exact cause. It is impractical for a first aid provider to distinguish among the many causes of abdominal pain because first aid will usually be similar regardless of the cause.

What to Do

1. Give water or clear fluids (fluids that you can see through, but **DO NOT** give alcohol or caffeine). Have the person slowly sip the fluids. Avoid solid foods.
2. Give the person an antacid (eg, Tums, Rolaids, Pepto-Bismol). If these fail, try a medication that helps stop stomach acid secretion (eg, Tagamet and Pepcid AC). If these fail, evacuate.
3. If practical, place a hot-water bottle against the person's abdomen, or have the person soak in a warm bath.

4. Be prepared for vomiting by keeping the person on their side (recovery position).
5. Have the person lie down with knees bent.
6. Evacuate if any of the following applies:
   - Pain is constant for more than 6 hours.
   - The person is unable to drink fluids.
   - The person is or might be pregnant.
   - Significant recent abdominal injury exists.
   - The abdomen is rigid and painful.
   - The abdomen is swollen.
   - More pain occurs after pressing your fingers on person's abdomen and suddenly releasing it.
   - There is bloody, blood-stained, or black stool or vomit.
   - The person has a fever.
   - There is light-headedness or fainting.
   - Pain began around the navel (belly button) and later moved to the lower right abdomen. This is a sign of appendicitis.

Nausea and Vomiting

Vomiting and nausea often occur with conditions such as mild acute mountain sickness, motion sickness, brain injury, intestinal viruses, food poisoning, eating or drinking too much, and emotional distress.

What to Do

1. Give small amounts of water or clear fluids (eg, sports drinks, clear soups) but **DO NOT** give alcohol or caffeine. Have the person slowly sip the fluids. Avoid solid foods. Later, if the person is

able to keep fluids down, offer carbohydrates (eg, bread, cereal, crackers, pasta) first. Avoid dairy products and meats for 48 hours.

2. Rest and avoid exertion until the person is able to eat solid foods easily.
3. Be prepared for vomiting.
4. Evacuate if any of the following applies:
   - Blood or brown, grainy material appears in vomit.
   - Constant abdominal pain.
   - Person faints when standing.
   - Person is unable to keep fluids down for more than 24 hours.
   - Person has severe projectile vomiting (vomit shoots out in large quantities).
   - Person suffered an abdominal injury.
   - Vomiting follows a recent head injury.

Diarrhea

Diarrhea is the frequent (usually more than four times per day) passage of loose, watery, or unformed stools. Let diarrhea run its course because bacteria or parasites are expelled and are not trapped in the intestines.

What to Do

1. Give water or clear fluids. Have the person slowly sip the fluids. This is the single most important treatment. Avoid solid foods. Later, give clear soups and bland foods (eg, toast, crackers, oatmeal).

2. Give a bismuth preparation (follow the label directions). It can turn the stool and tongue black. Those who are sensitive to aspirin, as well as children under 12 and teenagers, should not use it. If the person must be in control of their stools, over-the-counter medications will calm the bowel, reducing movement through the intestines.
3. Evacuate if any of the following applies:
   - Blood in stools that may appear black (keep in mind that bismuth preparations can cause black stools)
   - No improvement after 24 hours
   - Fever
   - Severe, constant abdominal pain
   - Severe dehydration

Constipation

Constipation is the passage of hard, dry stools occurring fewer than three times a week.

What to Do

1. Make sure the person drinks plenty of fluids (eight to ten 8-ounce glasses daily).
2. Have the person eat fiber (fresh or dried fruits, vegetables, or bran). Over-the-counter fiber products (Metamucil or Citrucel) can be used (follow label directions). **DO NOT** give a laxative.
3. Encourage the person to remain active.
4. If no improvement occurs, try caffeine or a stool softener.

5. Evacuate if any of the following applies:
   - Severe abdominal pain
   - Visibly swollen abdomen accompanied by pain
   - Fever
   - Vomiting

Abdominal Injuries

What to Look for	What to Do
Penetrating object	**DO NOT** remove a penetrating object. Stabilize the object against movement. **DO NOT** give the person anything to eat or drink. Evacuate immediately.
Protruding organs	**DO NOT** try to push protruding organs back into the abdomen. **DO NOT** touch organs. Cover them with a moist, clean dressing. **DO NOT** give the person anything to eat or drink. Evacuate immediately.
Hard blow to abdomen	Roll the person onto one side with the legs bent and expect vomiting. **DO NOT** give the person anything to eat or drink. Evacuate.

Alcohol and Drug Emergencies

Alcohol Intoxication

What to Look for	What to Do
■ Odor of alcohol ■ Unsteady, staggering gait ■ Slurred speech and inability to carry on a conversation ■ Nausea and vomiting ■ Flushed face	**1.** Monitor breathing. **2.** Check for injuries. **3.** Keep the person on their side.

Drugs

Drugs are classified according to their effects on the user.

What to Look for	What to Do
■ **Uppers** stimulate the central nervous system. Examples are amphetamines and cocaine. ■ **Downers** depress the central nervous system. Examples are barbiturates, tranquilizers, marijuana, and narcotics.	**1.** Monitor breathing, and if absent, give CPR. **2.** Check for injuries. **3.** Keep the person on their side. **4.** Evacuate. **5.** For an opioid overdose, ask others about the availability of an overdose kit (contains naloxone [Narcan]). It may be a nasal spray or an auto-injector.

Continues

What to Look for	What to Do
■ **Hallucinogens** alter the senses (eg, vision). Examples are LSD (lysergic acid diethylamide), mescaline, peyote, and PCP (phencyclidine, angel dust). Marijuana also has some hallucinogenic capabilities. ■ **Volatile chemicals** usually are inhaled and can seriously damage many body organs. Examples are paint solvents, gasoline, and spray paint.	

Warning

- **DO NOT** let an intoxicated or drugged person sleep on their back.
- **DO NOT** leave an intoxicated or drugged person alone.
- **DO NOT** try to handle a violent person by yourself—find a safe place, and call law enforcement officials.

Allergic Reactions (Severe)

Severe reactions to medications, food and food additives, insect stings, and plant pollen can be life threatening (called anaphylaxis).

What to Look for	What to Do
▪ Warm feeling followed by intense itching ▪ Skin flushes; face may swell ▪ Sneezing, coughing, wheezing ▪ Shortness of breath ▪ Tightness and swelling in the throat ▪ Tightness in the chest ▪ Increased heart rate ▪ Swelling of tongue, mouth, nose ▪ Blueness around lips and mouth ▪ Dizziness ▪ Nausea and vomiting	**1.** Monitor breathing, and if absent, give CPR. **2.** If the person has their own physician-prescribed epinephrine, help them use it. Inject at mid-thigh (can be given through clothing). About 20% require a second dose. **3.** If the person can swallow, give antihistamine (Benadryl)—note that it is not lifesaving because it takes too long to work, but can prevent further reactions. **4.** Evacuate immediately.

Altitude Illnesses

Going above 8,000 feet (2,500 meters) can produce one of several types of altitude illnesses. Altitude illnesses are caused by a prolonged lack of oxygen in the blood and tissues due to low air pressure at higher elevations **FIGURE 2**.

	AMS	HAPE	HACE
Elevation	Above 8,000 ft (2,438 m)	Usually above 10,000 ft (3,048 m)	Above 12,000 ft (3,658 m)
Time after ascent	Within several hours, up to 2 days later	3 to 4 days, possibly later	Within 24 hours, up to 7 days later
Cause and Symptoms	Symptoms of hypoxia: headache, sleep disturbance, fatigue, shortness of breath, dizziness, loss of appetite, nausea with or without vomiting	Symptoms of fluid in the lungs: shortness of breath, dry cough, mild chest pain, weakness, insomnia, rapid pulse, cyanosis, crackles (formerly known as rales), or gurgling sounds	Symptoms of increased fluid pressure in the brain: severe headache (unrelieved), vomiting, Cheynes-Stokes breathing (irregular breathing pattern that includes periods of apnea [no breathing]), ataxia (irregular gait or lack of coordination), unconsciousness
First aid	■ Stop ascending or return to a lower altitude. ■ Drink fluids. ■ Rest. ■ Take aspirin or ibuprofen according to package directions.	■ Descend at least 2,000 ft (610 m). ■ Seek professional medical attention. ■ **DO NOT** go down alone. ■ **DO NOT** delay descent.	■ Descend 4,000 ft (1,219 m) ■ Seek professional medical attention. ■ **DO NOT** go down alone. ■ **DO NOT** delay descent. ■ Give high-flow supplemental oxygen if available and you are trained.

	AMS	HAPE	HACE

	▪ Take acetazolamide.
	▪ If you are trained, give high-flow supplemental oxygen, if available.
		▪ If immediate descent is not possible:
		  ▪ Give high-flow supplemental oxygen if available and you are trained.
		  ▪ Use a portable hyperbaric chamber if available and you are trained.
			▪ Use a portable hyperbaric chamber if available and you are trained.

Notes: AMS = acute mountain sickness; HAPE = high-altitude pulmonary edema; HACE = high-altitude cerebral edema.

HAPE and HACE occur when reduced oxygen causes capillary leakage and body tissue swelling. Both conditions are life threatening.

Other Altitude-Related Illnesses

Pharyngitis and Bronchitis

Because of dry air, a sore throat and coughing may develop. The person should drink fluids, have an OTC antibiotic ointment applied in the nose, and suck hard candy or throat lozenges.

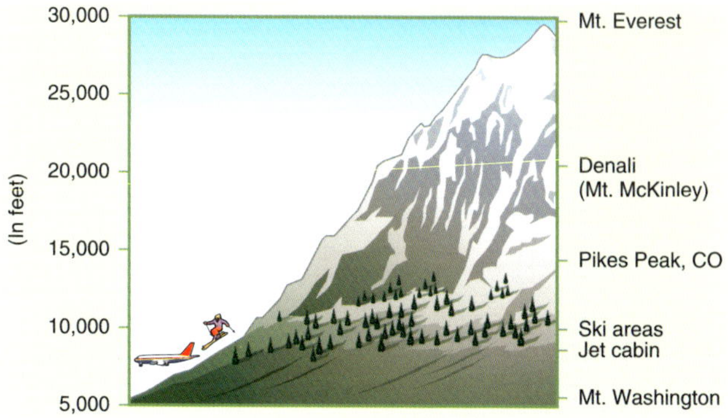

FIGURE 2 Various altitudes.

Peripheral Edema

Swelling of hands, ankles, and/or face (around the eyes) may appear at higher altitudes. If possible, raise the person's affected arms and/or legs. After descending or with acclimatization to higher altitudes, the swelling usually diminishes. Descend if signs of more serious altitude illnesses appear.

Arthropod Bites and Stings

Arthropods—including scorpions, spiders, centipedes, and ticks—are invertebrates with jointed legs and segmented bodies. Stinging insects cause more deaths than do venomous snakes **FIGURES 3–6**.

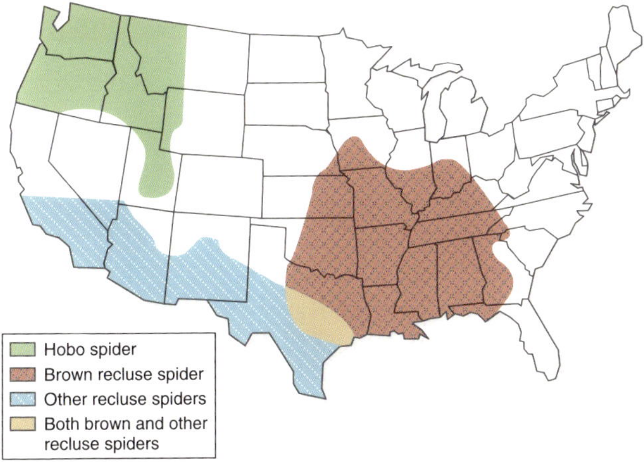

FIGURE 3 Map of spider range. Note that, with the exception of Alaska, black widow spiders are present across the United States.

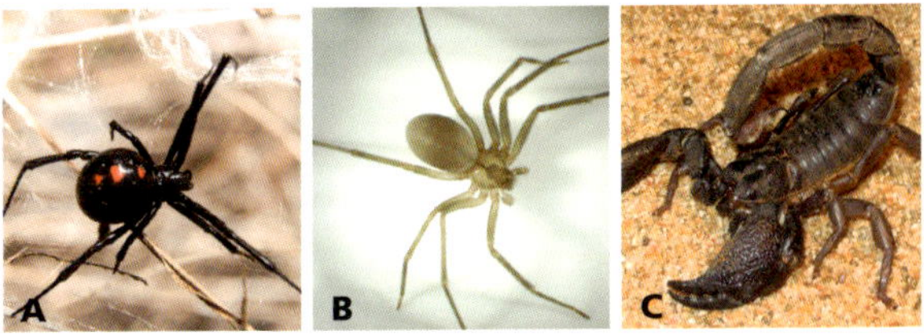

FIGURE 4 **A.** Black widow. **B.** Brown recluse. **C.** Scorpion.

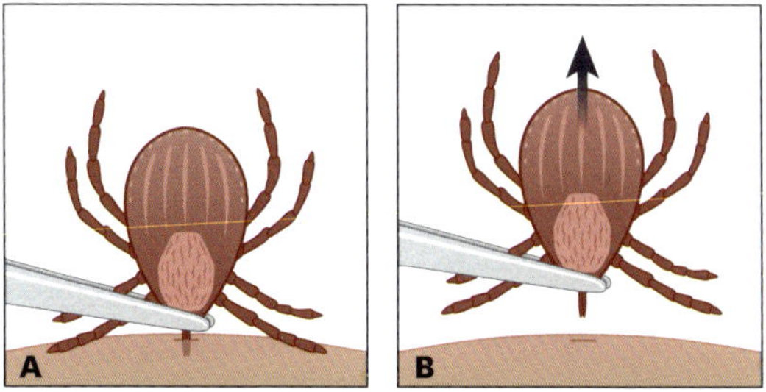

FIGURE 5 Removing a tick with tweezers. **A.** Grasp the tick as close to the skin as possible. **B.** Pull upward with steady, even pressure.

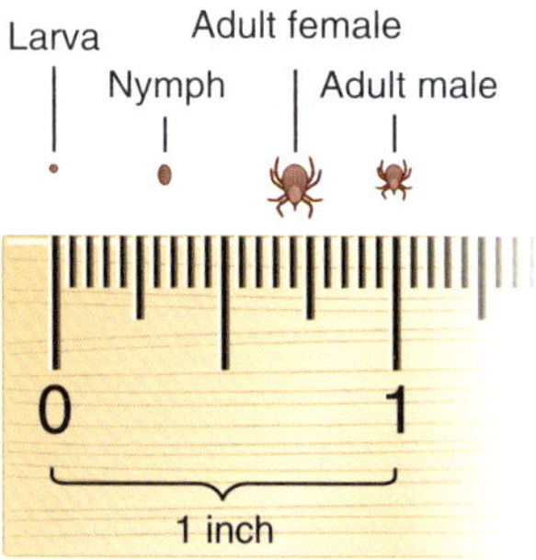

FIGURE 6 Approximate size of blacklegged tick (deer tick) at different life stages.

Arthropod	What to Look for	What to Do
Stinging insects ▪ Honeybee ▪ Bumblebee ▪ Hornet ▪ Yellow jacket ▪ Wasp ▪ Fire ants Those who have had a previous severe reaction should wear a medical alert ID tag and carry a physician-prescribed epinephrine kit.	▪ Usual reactions: instant pain, redness, itching. ▪ Worrisome reactions: hives, swollen lips/tongue, "tickle" in throat, wheezing. ▪ Life-threatening reactions: blue/gray skin color (in any skin tone), seizures, unresponsiveness, inability to breathe because of swollen vocal cords. ▪ About 60% to 80% of anaphylactic deaths are caused by person's inability to breathe because of swollen airway passages.	**1.** Look for a stinger, and if found, remove it as soon as possible (eg, brush off with your hand or scrape it with a fingernail or credit card). **DO NOT** use tweezers. Only bees leave their stinger embedded. **2.** Wash the area with soap and water. **3.** Apply an ice pack over the area. Baking soda paste may help except for wasp stings. **4.** Give pain medication. Apply hydrocortisone cream (1%) and give an antihistamine (Benadryl). **5.** For a severe allergic reaction, help the person self-administer epinephrine.
Widow spider bites Best known as the black widow, but the term "black widow" is inaccurate because only three of the five species of widow spiders are black; the others are brown and gray.	▪ May feel sharp pinprick followed by dull, numbing pain ▪ Two small fang marks seen as tiny red spots	**1.** Clean the bitten area with soap and water. **2.** Apply an ice pack to the area for up to 20 minutes. **3.** Give OTC pain medication. **4.** Evacuate immediately.

Continues

Arthropod	What to Look for	What to Do
Only adult females bite. They have a shiny, black abdomen with a red or yellow spot that is often in the shape of an hourglass, or white spots or bands on the abdomen.	■ Severe abdominal pain (bites on arm can produce severe chest pain, thus mimicking a heart attack) ■ Headache, chills, fever, heavy sweating, nausea, and vomiting ■ Most people never see the spider.	
Fiddle back spider bites Also known as brown recluse spider, violin spider, and brown spider.	■ Mild to severe pain occurs within 2 to 8 hours. ■ A blister develops within 48 to 72 hours, becomes red, and bursts. It takes on a "bull's-eye" appearance. ■ Nausea, vomiting, headache, and fever	**1.** Same as for black widow spider. **2.** If wound becomes infected, apply antibiotic ointment under sterile dressing. **3.** Evacuate.
Hobo spider bites Also known as the aggressive house spider.	Same as for fiddle back spiders.	Same as for fiddle back spiders.

Arthropod	What to Look for	What to Do
Tarantula spider bites They bite only when vigorously provoked or roughly handled. They can flick their hairs onto a person's skin.	■ Pain varies from mild to severe throbbing lasting up to 1 hour.	Same as for black widow spider. For hairs in the skin, remove with sticky tape, wash with soap and water, apply hydrocortisone cream (1%), and give antihistamine (Benadryl) and an OTC pain medication.
Scorpion stings In the United States, only the bark scorpion found in Arizona is potentially deadly—it is active from May through August.	■ Burning pain ■ Numbness or tingling occurs later.	**1.** Monitor breathing. **2.** Wash the area with soap and water. **3.** Apply an ice pack to the area. **4.** Give OTC pain medication. **5.** Apply dressing. **6.** Evacuate for severe reactions.
Centipede bites Do not confuse with millipedes, which cannot inject venom but can irritate the skin.	■ Burning pain ■ Inflammation ■ Mild swelling of lymph nodes	Most bites will get better without treatment. **1.** Clean the wound with soap and water. **2.** Apply an ice pack over the area. **3.** Give OTC pain medication. **4.** If symptoms persist, give antihistamine (Benadryl) or apply hydrocortisone cream (1%) on the bite site. **5.** Evacuate for severe reactions.

Continues

Arthropod	What to Look for	What to Do
Embedded tick Most ticks are harmless, but can carry diseases (ie, Lyme disease, Rocky Mountain spotted fever, Colorado tick fever, Tularemia, etc). If a tick is carrying a disease, the longer it stays embedded, the greater the chance that the disease will be transmitted.	■ No pain initially exists, and the tick can go unnoticed for days without detection. ■ Red area around tick means it has punctured skin and is feeding on person's blood. ■ If the tick is engorged with blood, it means there is an increased risk of disease transmission. ■ May cause rash, fever, and chills. ■ The bite varies from a small bump to extensive swelling and ulcer.	Ticks are difficult to remove. Partial removal can lead to infection. **1.** Use tweezers or a tick removal tool. Grasp the tick close to the skin and pull up, gently tenting the skin. Hold tension until the tick releases. **DO NOT** jerk or twist the tick. If the tick's mouth parts break off and remain in the skin, apply warm soaks and an OTC antibiotic ointment. **2.** Wash your hands and the area with soap and water. Apply alcohol gel to further disinfect the area. **3.** Apply an ice pack over the area. **4.** If tick was engorged, seek professional medical advice. If traveling in "tick country," consult with a physician for advice before the trip. **5.** Watch for signs of infection such as headache, fever, or rash appearing 3 to 30 days after the tick bite. If symptoms appear, seek professional medical advice.

Arthropod	What to Look for	What to Do
		Cautions about removing an embedded tick: ■ **DO NOT** use a hot match, fingernail polish, alcohol, petroleum jelly, or gasoline.
Chigger mite bites Bites can number in the hundreds.	■ Burning pain after several hours. ■ Local inflammation of the wound. ■ Small red welts appear. ■ Skin infection can result.	**1.** Wash the area with soap and water and rinse several times. **2.** Apply an ice pack over the area. **3.** Apply hydrocortisone cream (1%) or calamine lotion. **4.** Give an antihistamine (Benadryl).
Mosquito bites Human breath (contains carbon dioxide) and sweat attract mosquitoes.	■ Itching ■ Mild swelling	**1.** Wash the affected area with soap and water. **2.** Apply an ice pack over the area. **3.** Apply calamine lotion or hydrocortisone cream (1%) to decrease itching. **4.** For a person with numerous stings or a delayed allergic reaction, an antihistamine (Benadryl) every 6 hours or a physician-prescribed cortisone might be helpful.

Continues

Arthropod	What to Look for	What to Do
Fleas	■ Itching ■ Multiple bites, termed "breakfast, lunch, and dinner," are common.	**1.** Apply an ice pack over the area. **2.** Apply hydrocortisone cream (1%). **3.** Give an antihistamine (Benadryl).

Asthma

Asthma is a long-term lung condition that inflames and narrows the airways (tubes that carry air into and out of the lungs). The episodes can be occasional or often. Between episodes, the person has no trouble breathing. Asthma varies from one person to another, with symptoms ranging from mild to severe, and can be life threatening.

What to Look for	What to Do
■ Frequent coughing ■ Wheezing (whistling or squeaky sound during breathing) ■ Shortness of breath	**1.** Have the person sit in an upright position, leaning slightly forward. **2.** Encourage the person to sit and breathe slowly and deeply in through the nose and out through the mouth. **3.** Ask the person about any asthma medication they use. Most people with asthma usually have a doctor-prescribed quick-relief inhaler, also called a metered-dose inhaler or MDI.

What to Look for	What to Do
▪ Sitting in tripod position (leaning forward with hands on knees or other support, trying to breathe) ▪ Unable to speak in complete sentences without stopping to breathe	**4.** Help the person use the quick-relief inhaler: **a.** Remove the cap, shake the inhaler 10–15 times, and apply the spacer, if available. **b.** Ask the person to take a deep breath in and then breathe out all the way. **c.** Have the person hold the inhaler upright and between their index finger and thumb. **d.** Have the person put the inhaler or spacer mouthpiece in their mouth, above their tongue and between their teeth, then close their lips around it. **e.** Have the person start breathing in slowly and then press down on the inhaler once (to release the medication) while breathing in all the air they can, and then hold for 5–10 seconds with their mouth closed. **f.** Once the 5–10 seconds are up, tell the person to open their mouth and breathe out slowly. **g.** If the person needs another dose, wait 1 minute before repeating the above steps. **5.** Evacuate if: **a.** There is no improvement after using the medication or there is no rescue inhaler. **b.** Repeated attacks occur.

Continues

What to Look for	What to Do
	c. There is a severe and prolonged attack. **d.** The person struggles to breathe, talk, or stay awake. **e.** The person is unable to speak one or two words in one breath. **f.** The person's lips or fingernails turn blue. **g.** The person asks for professional medical care. **6.** **DO NOT** assume the person's condition is improving if wheezing is no longer heard.

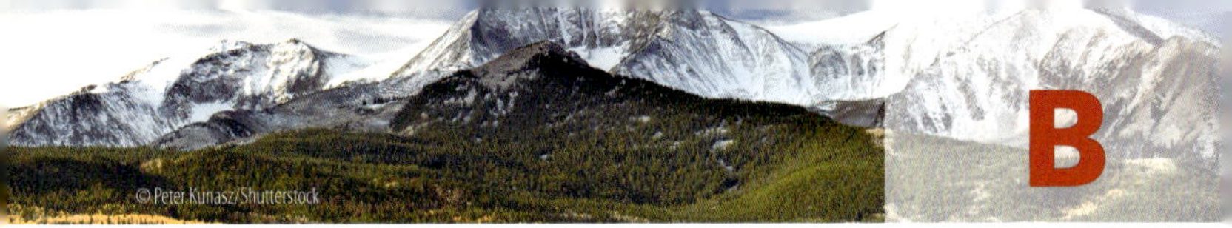

Bleeding and Wound Care

Bleeding Control

1. Expose the bleeding wound.
2. Avoid contact with blood by putting on disposable medical exam gloves. If gloves are unavailable, use a plastic bag, extra dressings, clean cloths, or have the person apply pressure with their own hand, if possible.
3. Stop the bleeding by placing a sterile dressing or clean cloth over the wound and pushing directly on the wound. This technique stops most bleeding. Remove a blood-soaked dressing and use a new dressing, then apply better aimed pressure on the wound **FIGURE 7**.
4. If bleeding fails to stop from the arm or leg, apply a manufactured tourniquet 2 to 3 inches above the wound. Apply a second tourniquet above and near the first one if bleeding continues.
5. If a manufactured tourniquet is not available, improvise and follow these directions:
    a. While making a tourniquet, continue applying pressure over the wound.

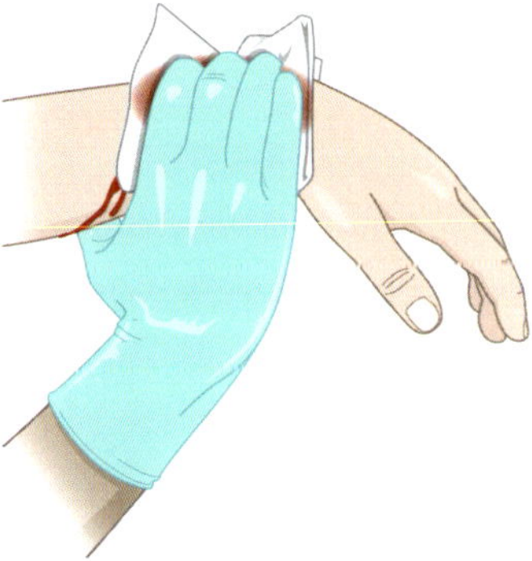

FIGURE 7 Applying pressure to a wound.

b. Make a tourniquet from a triangle bandage, neckerchief, wide roller bandage, or similar cloth into a long band about 3 to 4 inches wide and several layers thick. **DO NOT** use narrow materials (ie, wire, rope, or cord), which could cut into the skin.

c. Wrap the band around the arm or leg twice, placing it about 2 to 3 inches above the wound.

d. Tie the ends together over the wound.

e. Place a short (6 to 8 inches) and thick stick or similar object on the knot and then tie another knot over the stick (a square knot is best).

f. Twist the stick or similar object as you would a handle until bleeding stops. If a heartbeat can be felt at the wrist (for arm injuries) or behind the inside ankle knob (for a leg injury), the tourniquet is too loose. Secure the stick in place with another cloth band or tape to prevent it from unwinding.

g. Write "TQ" or "TK" (for tourniquet) and the exact time it was applied on a piece of adhesive tape and stick it to the person's forehead.

When using a tourniquet:

- **DO NOT** apply it anywhere except on an arm or leg—it does not work on the torso, head, neck, armpit, or groin.
- **DO NOT** apply it over any joint, but keep it as close to the wound as possible.
- **DO NOT** use narrow materials.
- Use wide padding under the tourniquet, if possible, to protect the tissues and help apply compression.
- **DO NOT** cover a tourniquet—leave it in view unless in a cold environment.
- **DO NOT** release a tourniquet unless professional medical care is more than 1 hour away. In this situation, **DO NOT** take it off; instead, release the tourniquet every 2 hours to quickly see if the bleeding has stopped or slowed to the point that a pressure bandage over the wound would be sufficient. While long-term tourniquet use may result in an amputation, it is better than death due to blood loss.

Hemostatic Dressing Use

When direct pressure is not effective, a tourniquet (TQ) is not available, a TQ is not effective, or a TQ cannot be applied (ie, the wound is on the abdomen, back, or chest), stuff or pack a hemostatic dressing into the wound and apply firm, direct pressure.

Wound Care

1. Clean the wound (this may restart bleeding):
   - **a.** For a shallow wound:
     - Wash inside and around the wound with soap and water.
     - Flush the inside of the wound with pressurized water that is clean enough to drink. This means using water from a faucet or an irrigation syringe. If using an irrigation syringe, flush 0.75 to 1 cup of water through the wound. Using a plastic bag with a small hole cut in it may be helpful. Pouring, soaking, or using a bulb syringe does not provide enough pressure to be effective but may be all that is available.
     - Cover the wound with a thin layer of an over-the-counter antibiotic ointment (eg, Neosporin or Polysporin). **DO NOT** use thiomersal (Merthiolate), merbromin (Mercurochrome), alcohol, iodine, or hydrogen peroxide because these are toxic to the tissues.
   - **b.** For a wound with a high risk for infection (eg, animal bite, very dirty or ragged wound, puncture wound), clean as best you can. Evacuate and seek professional medical help ASAP.

2. Cover shallow and high-risk wounds with a sterile dressing. Pack high-risk wounds with gauze dressings held in place by a bandage.
3. Seek professional medical help to:
   - Clean wounds at high risk for infection.
   - Close wide and gaping open wounds (sutures [stitches] are best placed within 6 to 8 hours after an injury) or to treat an underlying structure (eg, tendon, nerve) that is injured.
   - Receive a tetanus booster, if necessary.

When possible, scrub hands vigorously with soap and water before and after giving help. If water is unavailable, use an alcohol hand sanitizer gel.

Infected Wound

Any wound, large or small, can become infected. Proper cleaning can help prevent infections.

What to Look for	What to Do
▪ Swelling and redness around wound ▪ Feels warmer than surrounding area ▪ Throbbing pain ▪ Pus discharge	1. Soak the wound in warm water, or apply warm, wet packs over the infected wound. Separate the wound edges to allow pus to escape. 2. Apply an antibiotic ointment. 3. Change the dressings several times a day. 4. Give pain medication. 5. Evacuate and seek professional medical help if the wound becomes worse.

Blood Under a Nail

What to Look for

A fingernail or toenail has been crushed or smashed, causing the person unbearable pain due to blood collecting under the nail.

What to Do

1. Immerse the finger in ice or cold water or apply an ice pack with the hand elevated to reduce pain and swelling.
2. Relieve pressure under the injured nail by using one of the following methods:
   - Use the eye end of a sewing needle, unfolded paperclip, or similar metal object. Hold the needle or metal with pliers, and use a match or lighter to heat it until the metal is red-hot. Press the glowing end of the needle against the nail so it melts through. Little pressure is needed. The nail has no nerves, so this treatment is painless **FIGURE 8**.

   OR

   - Using a rotary action, carefully drill through the nail with the sharp point of a knife, large needle, or small drill bit. This method may be painful and takes more time.
3. Apply a dressing to absorb the draining blood and to protect the injured nail.
4. If necessary, evacuate.

What to Look for	What to Do
Anterior shoulder (95% of all shoulder dislocations) ■ Inability to touch the opposite shoulder with hand of injured arm ■ Arm held away from body ■ Extreme pain ■ Deformity when compared with opposite shoulder	**1.** Check heart rate at the wrist. Ask the person if they feel you lightly squeezing their fingers; ask them to wiggle their fingers unless injured. **2.** Use the simple hanging method with 5 to 10 pounds of weight strapped to the wrist and lower arm (takes up to 60 minutes to work). **FIGURE 13** **3.** After reduction, stabilize shoulder with arm sling **FIGURE 14.** **4.** Apply an ice pack.
Patella (kneecap) ■ The kneecap moved to the outside of knee joint (large bulge visible under skin) ■ Deformity when compared with opposite knee ■ Extreme pain	**1.** Slowly straighten the leg. **2.** You may need to push the kneecap back in place while straightening the leg. **3.** Splint with leg straight. The person can usually walk on an injured leg. **4.** Apply an ice pack.
Finger ■ Deformity when compared with the finger on the person's opposite hand ■ Inability to use	**1.** Hold the end of the finger, and pull it in the direction it is pointing **FIGURE 15**. **2.** While pulling, swing the finger back into normal alignment. You may have to hyperextend the joint first. **3.** Splint with "buddy taping" with fingers slightly bent and gauze between them **FIGURE 16**. **4.** Apply an ice pack.

Continues

What to Look for	What to Do
	Note: ■ Try reducing only once. ■ **DO NOT** try reducing joint at base of index finger or base of thumb (both require surgery).

Evacuate and seek professional medical help for any shoulder, finger, or kneecap dislocations that cannot be relocated, and any dislocations of the wrist, elbow, hip, knee, and ankle.

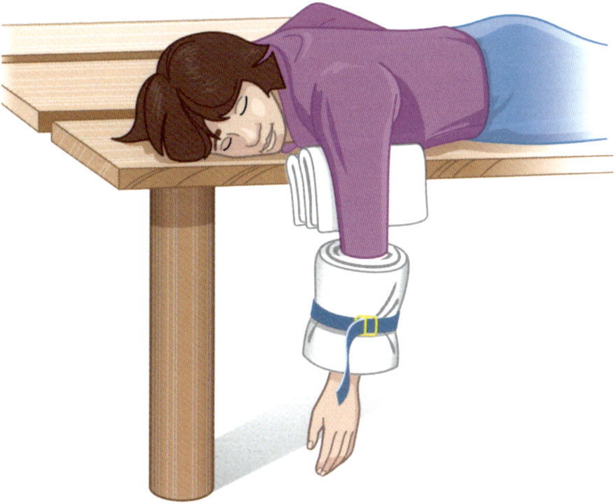

FIGURE 13 Simple hanging method to reduce a shoulder dislocation.

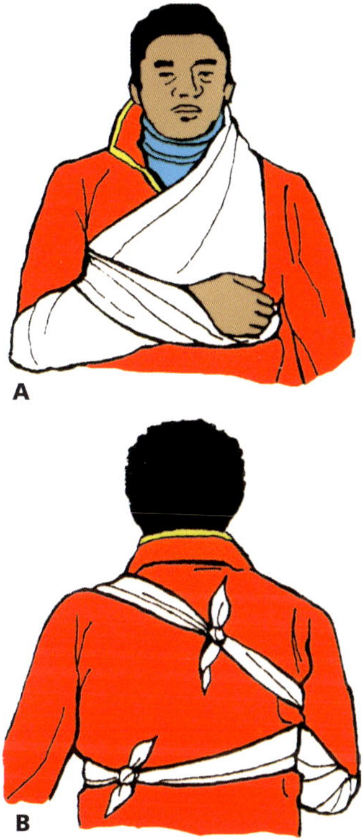

FIGURE 14 Sling and swathe (binder). **A.** Front. **B.** Back.

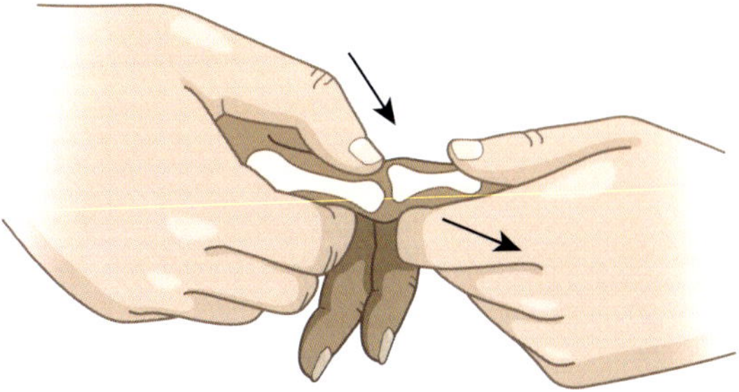

FIGURE 15 Reducing a finger dislocation.

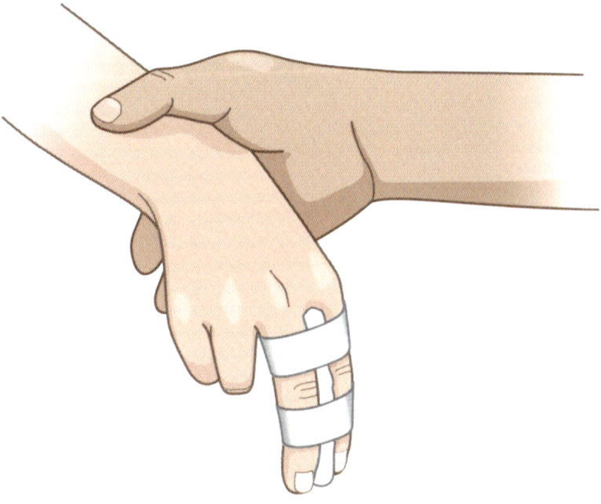

FIGURE 16 Splinting with buddy taping.

Ankle Injuries

What to Look for	What to Do
Any pain or tenderness in ankle and **1.** Bone tenderness along the back edge or tip of the ankle knob bone (malleolus), and **2.** Cannot bear weight and take four steps immediately after the injury or an hour later.	Suspect fractured ankle **1.** Treat with RICE. **2.** Stabilize against movement with a splint. **3.** Evacuate.
Any pain or tenderness in ankle and **1.** No bone tenderness along back edge or tip of ankle knob bone (malleolus) and **2.** Can bear weight and take four steps immediately after the injury and an hour later.	Suspect sprained ankle **1.** Treat with RICE. See **FIGURE 17** showing an elastic bandage being applied for compression. **2.** No evacuation is usually needed. **3.** **DO NOT** apply heat until 48 to 72 hours after injury.

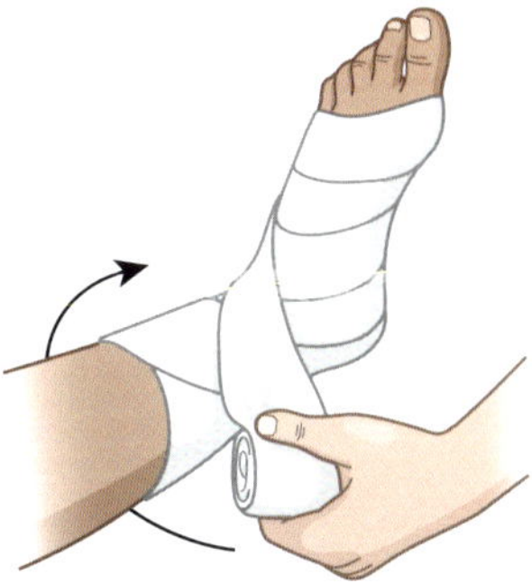

FIGURE 17 Apply an elastic bandage to compress a sprained ankle.

Knee Injuries

What to Look for	What to Do
Use one of these procedures to check for a knee injury: **1.** Pittsburgh Knee Rules If a blunt trauma or a fall caused the injury, plus one of the following: ■ Age $<$ 12 years or $>$ 50 years ■ Inability to walk four steps OR	**1.** Treat with RICE. **2.** Stabilize against movement with splint. **3.** Evacuate.

What to Look for	What to Do
2. Ottawa Knee Rules: ▪ Age > 55 years ▪ Tenderness at the patella (kneecap) ▪ Tenderness at head of fibula (bony knob on outside of knee ▪ Inability to flex knee to 90° ▪ Inability to bear weight and take four steps immediately after injury or an hour later	

Splinting Guidelines

All broken bones and dislocations should be stabilized before moving the person. When in doubt, apply a splint. Any device can be used to stabilize a broken bone or dislocation. The device can be improvised (eg, ski or hiking poles, canoe/kayak paddles, or pillow) or can be a commercial splint (eg, a SAM Splint). A self-splint is one in which the injured body part is tied to an uninjured part (eg, injured finger taped to adjacent finger, legs tied together, or arm tied to chest).

1. Cover open wounds with a dry, sterile dressing.
2. Check blood flow and nerves—for an arm, feel for a heartbeat at the wrist; for a leg, feel for a heartbeat behind the ankle knob on the inside. Ask the person if they feel you lightly squeezing their toes/fingers, and ask the person to wiggle their toes/fingers unless injured.

3. Determine what to splint by using the "Rule of Thirds." Imagine each long bone (eg, leg, arm) as being divided into thirds. If the injury is located in the upper or lower third of a long bone, assume that the nearest joint is injured. Therefore, the splint should extend to stabilize the bones above and below the joint. For a break of the middle third of a bone, stabilize the joints above and below the fracture. A broken arm, in addition to being splinted, should be placed in an arm sling and binder (ties arm to chest).
4. If two first aid providers are present, one should support the injured part to minimize movement until splinting is finished.
5. If possible, place splint materials on both sides of the injured part, especially when two bones are involved (eg, radius and ulna, tibia and fibula) to prevent bone rotation, which can produce pain and additional injury.
6. Apply splints firmly, but not tight enough to affect blood flow. Pad splints with clothing or other material for comfort.
7. Try to straighten a fracture only in remote locations and if one or both of the following exists: (1) an extremity is badly deformed and/or (2) no heartbeat can be felt in the injured extremity.
   DO NOT move a suspected injured spine or replace a dislocation, *except* anterior shoulder, kneecap, and finger dislocations.

Muscle Injuries

What to Look for	What to Do
▪ Sudden muscle pain ▪ A muscle, often the calf muscle, that feels hard because of the muscle contraction ▪ Often residual discomfort for a few hours	Suspect a muscle cramp (spasm). Try one or more of these to relax the muscle: **1.** Have the person gently stretch the affected muscle. **2.** Press on the muscle. **3.** Apply an ice pack to the muscle. **4.** For a calf muscle cramp only, have the person pinch the upper lip hard (an acupressure technique). **5.** Drink lightly salted cool water ($1/4$ teaspoon salt in 1 quart of water) or commercial sports drinks.
▪ A blow to a muscle ▪ Swelling ▪ Tender and painful ▪ Black and blue mark appears hours later	Suspect a muscle bruise (contusion). Use the RICE procedures.
▪ Occurs during physical activity ▪ Sharp pain ▪ Very tender ▪ Cannot use injured part ▪ Stiffness and pain when muscle is used	Suspect muscle strain (pull). Use the RICE procedures.

Evacuate and seek professional medical help for these injuries ASAP:

- A broken bone or dislocation with an open fracture
- No heartbeat felt in the extremity
- Suspected spinal cord injury
- Heavy blood loss
- Severe deformity affecting blood flow and/or sensation

Burns

1. Stop the burning! If clothing is on fire, have the person roll on the ground using the "stop, drop, and roll" method. Smother the flames with a blanket, or douse the person with water. Remove clothing and all jewelry, especially rings, from the burn area. If it is a chemical burn, wash with large quantities of water. Dry chemicals should be brushed off before flushing with large amounts of water.
2. Check and monitor breathing if the person breathed heated air or was in an explosion.
3. Determine the depth of the burn. This is difficult but helps determine what first aid to give.
4. Determine the size of the burn by using the "Rule of the Hand." The person's hand (includes palm, closed fingers, and thumb) equals about 1% of the person's total body surface area (TBSA).
5. Determine which parts of the body are burned. Burns on the face, hands, feet, and genitals are more severe than burns on other body parts.

What to Look for	What to Do
First-degree burn (superficial) ■ Redness ■ Mild swelling ■ Tenderness ■ Pain	**1.** Immerse the burned area in cold water, or apply a wet, cold cloth until pain-free both in and out of the water. If cold water is unavailable, use any cold liquid available. **DO NOT** apply ice, ice water, or salt water. **2.** Give ibuprofen (for children or teenagers, give acetaminophen). **3.** Have the person drink as much water as possible without becoming nauseous. **4.** Keep burned arm or leg raised and remove any jewelry. **5.** After burn has been cooled, apply aloe vera gel or an inexpensive moisturizer. First-degree burns do not need to be covered.
Small second-degree burn of less than 20% TBSA (partial-thickness) ■ Blisters ■ Swelling ■ Weeping of fluids ■ Severe pain	**1.** Follow same procedures (steps 1 through 4) as for a first-degree burn, with these additions: **2.** After burn has been cooled, apply thin layer of antibacterial ointment (eg, Bacitracin or Neosporin). **3.** **DO NOT** break any blisters. **4.** Cover burn with a dry, nonsticking, sterile dressing or a clean cloth.
Large second-degree burn of more than 20% TBSA (partial-thickness burn)	**1.** Follow steps 2 through 4 of first-degree burn care. **DO NOT** apply cold because it may cause hypothermia. **2.** **DO NOT** break any blisters. **3.** Evacuate.

Continues

What to Look for	What to Do
Third-degree burn (full-thickness) ■ Dry, leathery, gray colored, or charred skin	1. Cover burn with a dry, nonsticking, sterile dressing or clean cloth. 2. **DO NOT** apply cold. 3. **DO NOT** apply gel or ointment. 4. Evacuate.

Evacuation

Most burns are superficial and small partial-thickness burns, which rarely need medical help. Large partial-thickness and all full-thickness burns, burned airways, and circumferential burns (completely around body part) need evacuation ASAP.

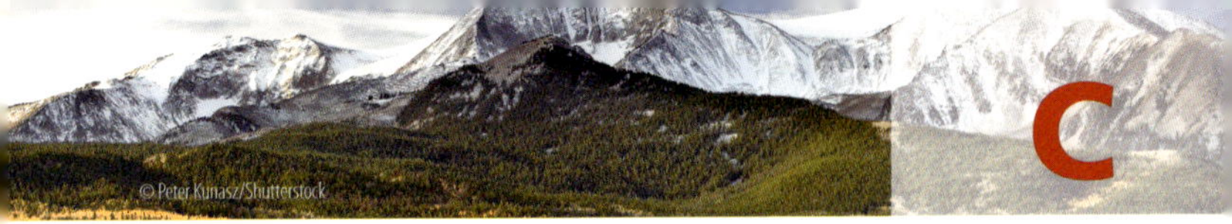

© Peter Kunasz/Shutterstock

Cardiac Arrest (Heart Stops)

CPR (Cardiopulmonary Resuscitation)

For a motionless person, use the mnemonic **RAB-CAB** to remember what to do. Start as soon as possible!

RAB

R = Responsive? Tap shoulder and shout, "Are you OK?"

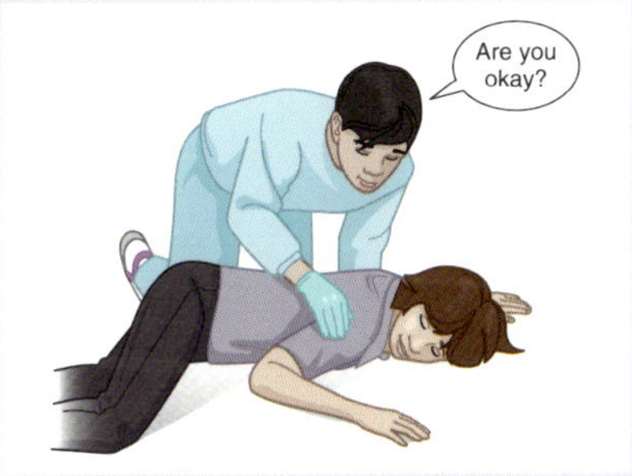

© Jones & Bartlett Learning.

Continues

If...	Then...
Unresponsive	Go to step **A = Activate**.

A = Activate EMS by asking another person(s) to go or call for help by using a mobile phone, satellite phone, or radio. A whistle can attract nearby people's attention who might be able to help.

If...	Then...
Alone	**For adult:** Immediately try calling for help and get AED (Automated External Defibrillator), if available. Then, return to the person to attach and use AED. **For child or infant:** Call for help after 5 cycles (2 minutes) of CPR.
Bystander or another rescuer is available	Send them to call for help or get help and AED, if available.

B = Breathing? Check for no breathing or only gasping. Observe the person from neck to waist for movement (rise and fall) for 5–10 seconds.

If...	Then...
Unresponsive and breathing normally	Place the person onto their side and monitor breathing.

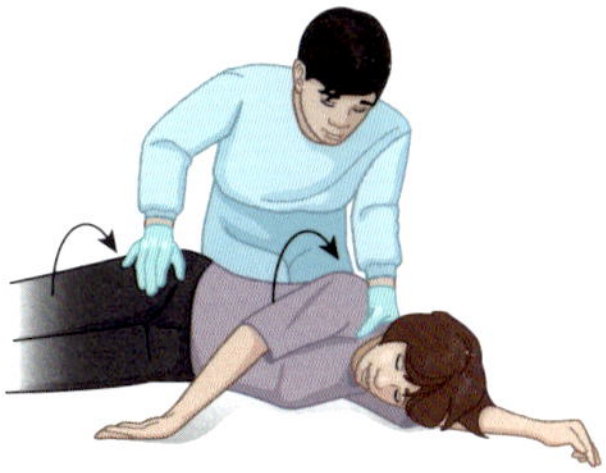

If...	Then...
Unresponsive and not breathing or only gasping	CPR is needed. Go to step **C = Compressions**.

CAB

C = Chest compressions. Push hard and fast.

Where to place hands?

For adult: Use 2 hands. Place heel of one hand on the center of the person's chest and on the lower half of their breastbone. Place your other hand on top of the first one with your fingers interlocked. Hold your fingers off the person's chest and point them directly away from you. **DO NOT** cross your hands.

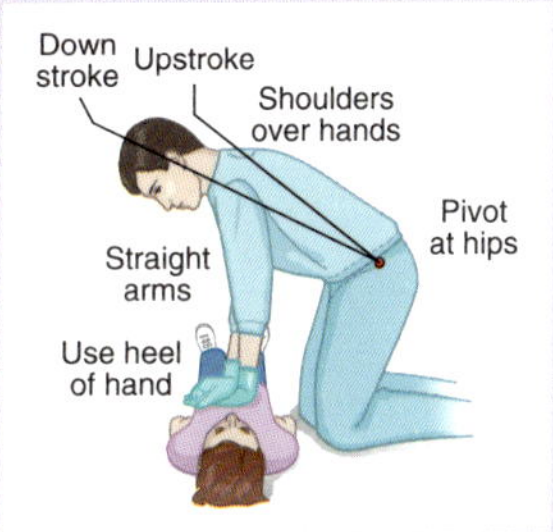

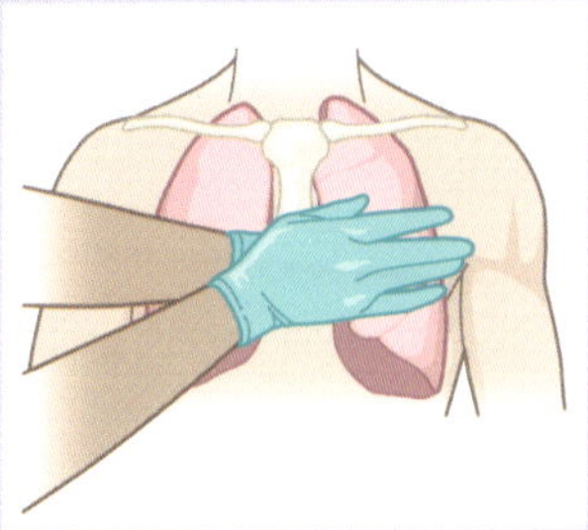

Continues

For child: Depending on the person's size and your own, use 1 or both hands in the same place as for an adult.

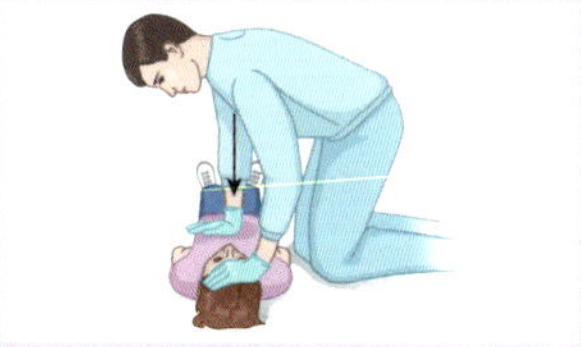

For infant: Place both thumbs on lower breastbone, both touching the imaginary nipple line and fingers encircling around the infant's back and chest.

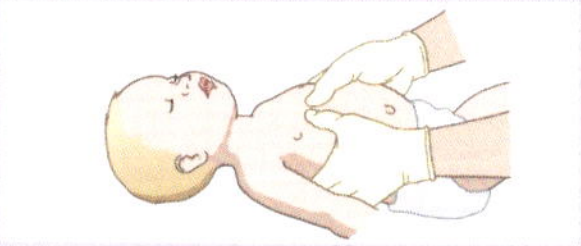

How deep?

Push hard!

For adult: Push straight down on chest at least 2 inches (5 cm).

For child: About 2 inches (5 cm) (about 1/3 depth of the chest).

For infant: About 1.5 inches (4 cm) (about 1/3 depth of the chest).

Allow chest to come back up to its normal position after each compression.

How fast?

Push fast!

Push chest at same beat of the Bee Gee's song, "Stayin' Alive." Count at fast rate: "1, 2, 3, 4 . . . 30. "This is at the rate of at least 100 to 120 compressions per minute.

How many?

Give 30 compressions without interruption unless AED arrives. If AED becomes available, use immediately.

A = Airway open. Open airway by tilting head back and lifting chin.

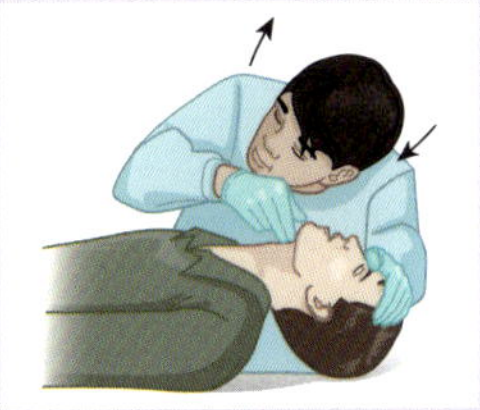

© Jones & Bartlett Learning.

B = Breaths. Give 2 normal breaths (1 second each) that make chest rise. Take a normal breath for yourself after each given breath.

For adult and child: Pinch the person's nose shut and make airtight mouth-to-mouth seal. Use CPR mask if available.

For infant: Cover mouth and nose with your mouth. If this does not work, try either mouth-to-mouth or mouth-to-nose.

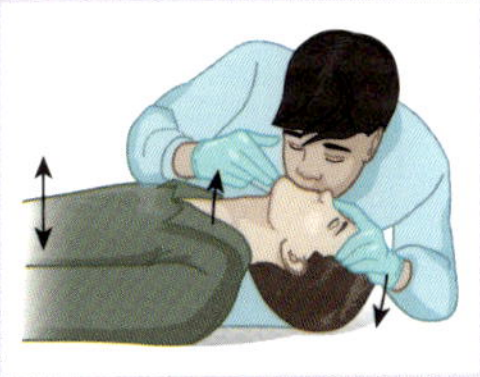

© Jones & Bartlett Learning.

Continues

If...	Then...
2 breaths make chest rise	Continue CPR: ■ 30 chest compressions (push hard and fast). ■ 2 breaths (1 second each). Take a regular breath, not a deep breath, for yourself between the 2 breaths. ■ Continue 30:2 compression to breath ratio until AED arrives and is ready to use, or until trained person takes over. ■ **DO NOT** stop to check for breathing until after 5 cycles of compressions and breaths.
First breath does not make chest rise; the airway may be blocked.	Retilt head, give a second breath ■ If second breath does not make chest rise, continue CPR. Each time the airway is opened to give a breath, look for an object in the person's mouth and, if found, remove it.
Continue CPR until ■ Person begins breathing ■ Trained rescuer(s) take over ■ AED arrives and is used ■ You are physically exhausted and unable to continue ■ Scene becomes unsafe	

Defibrillation

- Use AED as soon as possible.
- Expose chest, turn on AED, and attach pads following the manufacturer's direction for pad placement.
- Follow voice directions.

If...	Then...
If no shock advised	Resume CPR immediately (evaluate again by AED after 5 sets of 30 compressions and 2 breaths).
If shock advised	**DO NOT** touch the person. Give 1 shock or shocks advised by AED. Resume CPR immediately starting with compressions.

Hands-Only (Compression-Only) CPR

What to Look for	What to Do
If you see an adult or teen suddenly collapse and you: ▪ Are unable or unwilling to make mouth-to-mouth contact, ▪ Do not have a mouth-to-barrier device, or ▪ Are untrained in CPR.	1. **DO NOT** use hands-only CPR on an infant. Infants require rescue breaths. 2. Check the person for gasping or no breathing. 3. Ask another person(s) to go or call for help. 4. Push center of chest hard and fast (faster than 1 per second or use the beat of the Bee Gees' song "Stayin' Alive"). 5. Continue chest compressions until help arrives or as long as possible. If you get tired, switch with someone else (this may be every 2 minutes or 100 compressions).

CPR in Remote Locations

After cardiac arrest, a person's heart activity must be restored within a short time (most require medical help) for survival; thus, CPR is seldom successful in remote locations. Nevertheless, you should start CPR when breathing stops.

If any of the following conditions* are present, **DO NOT** start CPR:

- The environment is unsafe and dangerous to rescuers.
- Signs of death (eg, rigor mortis or stiff, rigid muscles)
- Obvious lethal injury (eg, decapitation)
- Documented do-not-resuscitate orders exist.
- Person has a rigid frozen chest.
- Known time from incident to resuscitation is too long (30 minutes since heart stopped, more than 1 hour after submersion in water).

If...	Then...
CPR is started in a remote location	Continue CPR until: ■ The person recovers. ■ Rescuers are too exhausted to continue. ■ Another rescuer takes over. ■ Scene becomes unsafe and rescuers become endangered. ■ AED is ready to use. ■ A physician tells you to stop. ■ The person does not respond to 30 minutes of resuscitation efforts (see the following list for exceptions).

If...	Then...
CPR is given for 30 minutes without success	Stop CPR. Exceptions when CPR should be given longer than 30 minutes: ■ Cool-water immersion of less than 1 hour ■ Avalanche burial ■ Hypothermia (in these instances, take 30 to 45 seconds to feel for a neck pulse before starting CPR) ■ Lightning strike

AED (Automated External Defibrillator)

Over 70% of those experiencing cardiac arrest are in ventricular fibrillation (ineffective heart muscle contractions). Early defibrillation is the single most important factor in saving lives from sudden cardiac arrest. CPR alone will seldom reverse cardiac arrest, but it does buy time by allowing an AED to arrive and be applied. Most remote locations will not have an AED readily available due to its weight, bulk, and cost. In urban areas, using CPR and an AED can save lives, but in remote locations, this combination will usually not revive a person unless there is fast access to an EMS system, most people will die. Because of these limitations, it is important to know when to start and stop giving CPR.

Give CPR until an AED arrives and is ready to use. Before using an AED, check for water or puddles around the person. Most AEDs use the same steps for adults, children, and infants:

1. Turn on the AED.
2. Attach the pads (as shown on the pads) on the person's bare, dry chest. If needed, plug the cables into the AED.
3. Stay clear of the person. Make sure no one, including you, is touching the person. Say, "Clear!"
4. Allow the AED to analyze the heart rhythm (push the "analyze" button, if necessary).
5. The AED prompts one of two actions: (a) stay clear and press the shock button if advised to deliver a shock, or (b) do not shock but give CPR starting with chest compressions with the pads staying in place.
6. After any one of the three actions, give 5 cycles of CPR (takes about 2 minutes when the AED says to stop to analyze heart rhythm), unless the person moves, begins to breathe, or wakes up.
7. Repeat steps 3 through 6 until the person starts to move, wakes up, or begins to breathe, or if more highly trained rescuers take over.

Chest Injuries

Chest injuries can involve broken bones, penetrating injuries, and open or closed wounds.

For all chest injuries, examine for the following:

- DOTS: deformity, open wounds, tenderness, and swelling.
- Abnormal breathing rate and/or sounds (ie, gurgling).
- Guarding (protecting an area during moving or touching).

Rib Fractures

What to Look for	What to Do
The following usually occur along the side of the chest: ▪ Sharp pain when the person takes deep breaths, coughs, or moves ▪ Person is holding (guarding) the area, trying to reduce pain ▪ Tenderness when touched ▪ Shallow breathing due to pain that occurs from normal or deep breathing ▪ Bruising of skin over the injury	**1.** Help the person find a comfortable position. **2.** Stabilize chest by: **a.** Having the person hold a pillow or other similarly soft material against the area, or **b.** Placing arm on the injured side in a sling and binder (swathe) if necessary for pain control **3.** **DO NOT** apply tight bandages around the chest. **4.** Give pain medication. **5.** Have the person cough and take deep breaths, even if it hurts, a few times every hour to prevent pneumonia. **6.** Evacuate and seek professional medical help.

Flail Chest

A flail chest happens when several ribs in the same area are broken in more than one place.

What to Look for	What to Do
▪ Area over the injury may move in a direction opposite to that of the rest of the chest wall during breathing.	**1.** Stabilize chest by: **a.** Placing a pillow or similarly soft material against area or arm on the injured side in a sling and binder (swathe) and

Continues

What to Look for	What to Do
■ Very painful and difficult breathing ■ Bruising of skin over the injury ■ Same as for Rib Fractures	**b.** Placing the person on their injured side with a blanket or similarly soft material underneath them. **2.** **DO NOT** apply tight bandages around the chest. **3.** Evacuate and seek professional medical help.

Penetrating Object in Chest

What to Look for	What to Do
■ Usually easy to see impaled object	**1.** Stabilize object in place with bulky dressings or clothes. **DO NOT** try to remove the object. **2.** Evacuate and seek professional medical help.

Open Chest Wound

What to Look for	What to Do
■ Blood bubbling out of a chest wound during exhalation ■ Sucking sound heard during inhalations	**1.** Open chest wounds require immediate evacuation to a medical facility. **2.** If bleeding does not occur, leave the wound exposed to air without a dressing or any airtight material.

What to Look for	What to Do
	3. If bleeding occurs, apply direct pressure with a dry gauze dressing to control bleeding. If the dressing becomes blood-soaked, replace it to avoid trapping air in the chest, which can result in death. **4.** Lean or lay the person on the injured side. **5.** Evacuate and seek professional medical help.

Chest Pain

What to Look for	What to Do
Muscle or rib pain from physical activity or injury	**1.** Have the person rest. **2.** Apply an ice pack to the affected area. **3.** Give pain medication.
Respiratory infection (bronchitis, pleuritis, pneumonia) ▪ Cough ▪ High fever and shaking chills, which are a sign of bacterial infection ▪ Sore throat ▪ Production of thick green or yellow sputum is a sign of bacterial infection.	**1.** Antibiotics are usually needed for bacterial infections and may be given if available. **2.** Antibiotics do not work for viral infections. **3.** Give fluids and pain medications. **4.** Evacuate and seek professional medical care if the person is worsening or having difficulty breathing.

Continues

What to Look for	What to Do
Indigestion ■ Belching ■ Heartburn ■ Nausea ■ Sour taste	1. Give antacids.
Angina pectoris (chest pain lasting less than 10 minutes)	1. Have the person rest. 2. Ask the person if they take any chest pain medication for a known heart condition, such as nitroglycerin, and help them take it. 3. Evacuate and seek professional medical help.
Heart attack (see *Heart Attack* section) ■ Chest pain in center of chest ■ Sweating ■ Light-headedness ■ Nausea or vomiting ■ Numbness, aching, or tingling in the arm ■ Shortness of breath ■ Weakness or fatigue	1. Have the person sit, with knees raised, and lean against a stable support (ie, fence post, tree trunk). Try to keep the person calm. **DO NOT** allow them to walk. 2. Loosen any tight clothing. 3. Ask if the person takes any chest pain medication for a known heart condition, such as nitroglycerin, and help them take it. 4. If the person is alert, able to swallow, and not allergic to aspirin, help the person take one adult aspirin (325 mg) or four low-dose aspirins (81 mg each). Pulverize or have the person crunch them with their teeth before swallowing for faster results. 5. Monitor breathing. If the person becomes unresponsive and stops breathing, begin CPR (see *Cardiac Arrest* section for CPR). 6. Evacuate and seek professional medical help immediately.

Choking

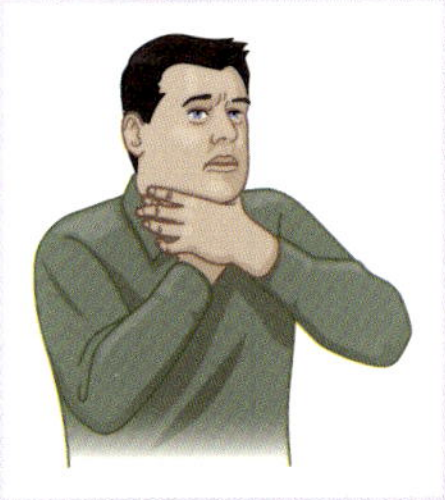

© Jones & Bartlett Learning.

1. Check the person for choking. Ask "Are you choking? Can you speak to me?" A choking person may be clutching the neck with one or both hands (this is the universal choking sign). They may also point to their mouth. A choking person cannot breathe, talk, cry, or cough.

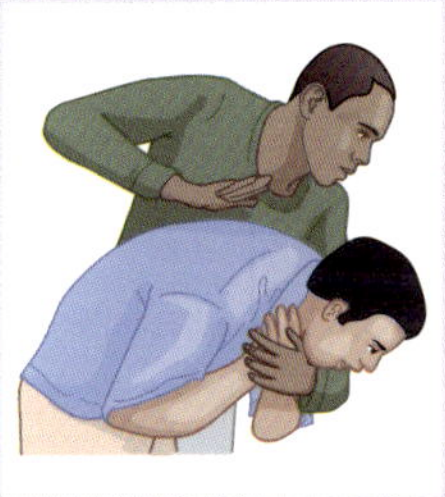

© Jones & Bartlett Learning.

2. Give 5 hard back blows:
   a. Stand behind the person and slightly to one side. Reach across the person's chest by wrapping one arm either over the person's arm or under their armpit. Place the palm of that hand on the person's upper chest or shoulder, leaving your other hand free.
   b. Have the person bend at the waist to a 90° angle. **DO NOT** keep them in a vertical position.
   c. With your fingertips up, use the heel of your hand to firmly strike the person between their shoulder blades.

Continues

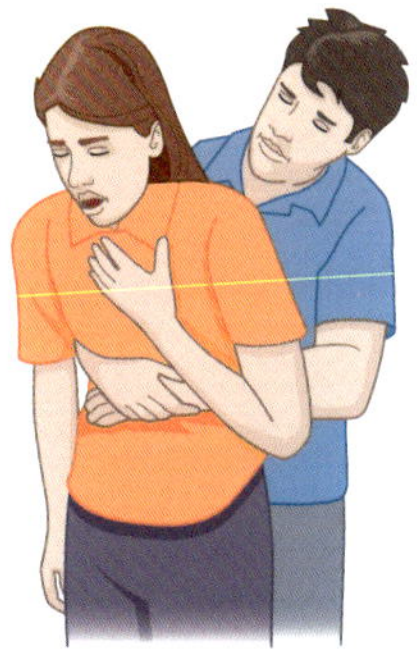

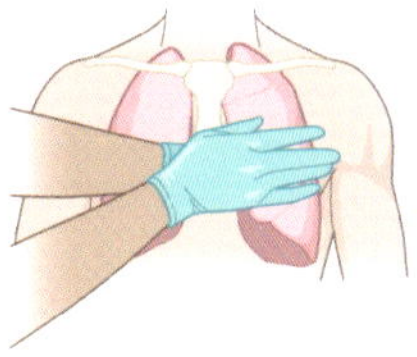

3. If 5 back blows do not dislodge the object, give up to 5 abdominal thrusts (or chest thrusts for a person who is pregnant or very large):
   a. Stand behind a choking adult or kneel behind a choking child. Wrap your arms around the person's waist and locate the navel with your fingers.
   b. Make a fist with one hand and place the thumb side of that hand just above the person's navel.
   c. Grasp your fist with the other hand and thrust your fist into the person's abdomen with a quick, inward and upward motion.
   d. If object is not dislodged after 5 thrusts, give 5 back blows. Continue by alternating with 5 back blows and 5 abdominal thrusts until the object is forced out or the person becomes unresponsive.
4. If the person becomes unresponsive and collapses onto ground, begin CPR. After 30 compressions and each time you open the airway to give breaths, look for an object in the throat, and if seen, remove it.

5. For an infant who is choking, give 5 separate and distinct back blows followed by 5 separate and distinct chest thrusts. Give the 5 chest thrusts in the same way you would for CPR chest compressions described above. Continue 5 back blows and 5 chest thrusts until the object is dislodged or the infant becomes unresponsive. If the infant becomes unresponsive, give CPR but before giving 2 breaths, look into the mouth for an object; if seen, remove it.

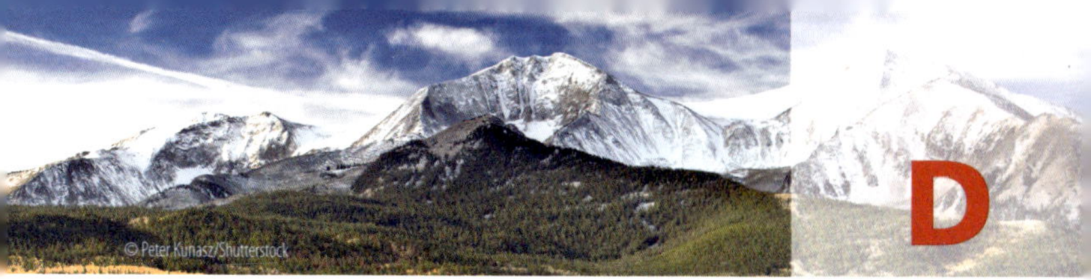

Diabetic Emergencies

When the body has too much sugar (glucose) present in the blood, the person is said to have diabetes mellitus, or simply "diabetes."

Before going into remote locations, a person with diabetes should tell the group's leader that they have diabetes; discuss the planned trip with their physician; and carry adequate supplies of necessary medicines and other equipment (ie, insulin, syringes, needles, pills, glucometer with fresh battery, lancets, plenty of test strips, etc), including extra supplies for emergencies. An injectable medication called glucagon can raise blood sugar in an emergency. Another group member might agree to carry these extra supplies, and should be taught how to test blood sugar and inject glucagon in case the person with diabetes becomes incapacitated. Insulin and glucagon should be protected from the cold (in an inside pocket in cold weather) or heat (in a closed vacuum bottle or buried in the pack). A person with diabetes should also carry extra food and snacks, so that they do not have to rely on others in the group if food is needed quickly **FIGURE 18**.

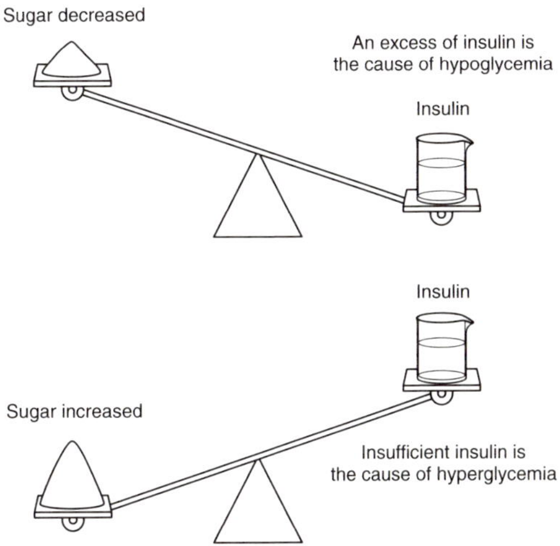

FIGURE 18 Diabetic emergencies are caused by either too much or too little insulin.

Hypoglycemia (Blood Sugar Too Low)

Hypoglycemia is a life-threatening emergency caused when the person with diabetes does any one of the following:

- Takes too much insulin (rapidly depletes sugar)
- Does not eat (reduces sugar intake)
- Overexerts themself or exercises (uses sugar faster)
- Vomits (empties stomach of sugar)

Most people with diabetes monitor their blood glucose levels as often as four times a day to maintain thc proper levels and to prevent a diabetic emergency. Hypoglycemia can rapidly progress to a life-threatening situation.

What to Look for	What to Do
■ Responsive and can swallow ■ Medical identification tag ■ Shaky, trembling ■ Cold, clammy, or moist skin ■ Confused ■ Light-headed or dizzy ■ Sudden hunger ■ Nauseated ■ Tingling or numbness in the lips, tongue, or cheeks ■ Heavy sweating	The person may be able to tell what is wrong and what to do. **1.** If the person has a blood glucose monitor and is capable, have them check their blood glucose level—it's the only sure way to know if a person is experiencing low blood sugar. **2.** For hypoglycemia, use the following procedure, but only when: ■ Testing is not possible and low blood sugar is suspected. ■ Testing shows a low blood sugar (glucose) level (below 70 mg/dL). ■ Profuse sweating or shaking occurs in a person known to have diabetes. **3.** The procedure is as follows (if the person can swallow): ■ Have the person eat 15 to 20 g of sugar. ■ If available, three to five glucose tablets is preferred (as directed on the label). ■ If glucose tablets are not available, give any form of sugar such as glucose gel tube (as directed on label); 4 ounces (1/2 cup) of fruit juice (eg, orange, apple); 4 ounces (1/2 cup) of regular soda (not diet); 3 to 5 teaspoons of table sugar or honey; or hard candies, jellybeans, gumdrops (check the food label for how many to consume). ■ Wait 10 to 15 minutes for the sugar to get into the blood.

What to Look for	What to Do
	▪ Recheck the blood glucose level, or if there is no monitor, look for improvement. ▪ If the blood glucose level is still low or no monitor was used and the person still has symptoms of low blood sugar, give the person an additional 15 g of sugar. **4.** If the person has no gag reflex and cannot swallow, **DO NOT** give anything by mouth. **5.** If there is no improvement or they cannot be given sugar, evacuate immediately. *Notes:* ▪ Young children usually need less than 15 g of carbohydrates to fix a low blood sugar level (eg, infants, 6 g; toddlers 8 g, small children 10 g). ▪ For a suspected hypoglycemic and uncooperative child who rejects swallowing a form of glucose, glucose placed under the tongue (sublingual) can be attempted. ▪ Many people may want to eat as much as they can until they feel better. This can cause blood sugar levels to shoot way up. Using the procedure described here can help avoid this (high blood sugar levels).
Severe hypoglycemia suspected: ▪ Staggering, slurred speech, and not following simple commands	**1.** If there is no improvement, seek professional medical help immediately. **2.** If not breathing, begin CPR. **3.** If breathing, roll them onto their side (recovery position) and monitor breathing. **4.** **DO NOT** give food or fluids. **5.** If unsure which diabetic condition (low blood sugar or high blood sugar) exists, give sugar. **DO NOT** give insulin.

What to Look for	What to Do
■ Unable to swallow ■ Seizures ■ Unresponsiveness	

Hyperglycemia (Blood Sugar Too High)

This condition occurs when a person with diabetes has too much sugar in their blood. Several conditions can cause this (ie, insufficient insulin, overeating, illness, inactivity, stress, or a combination of these factors). Hyperglycemia in remote locations is rarely encountered unless a person with diabetes is stranded and has either lost or run out of their diabetes medication. Hyperglycemia can be fatal if not treated within 24 hours.

What to Look for	What to Do
■ Medical identification tag ■ Gradual onset (hours to days) because some sugar is still reaching the brain ■ Drowsiness ■ Extreme thirst ■ Very frequent urination ■ Warm, red, dry skin ■ Vomiting	**1.** Give frequent, small sips of water if the person with diabetes can swallow. **2.** If possible, have a family member check their blood sugar level. If uncertain whether the person with diabetes has a high or low blood sugar level, and they are responsive and able to swallow, use the procedures for giving sugar, as described previously. The extra sugar will not cause any significant harm in the person experiencing hyperglycemia.

What to Look for	What to Do
▪ Fruity breath odor (has also been described to be like nail polish remover) ▪ Heavy breathing ▪ Eventual unresponsiveness	3. **DO NOT** give insulin unless the person with diabetes can self-administer it. 4. Call 9-1-1 as soon as possible.

Drowning (Submersion/Immersion)

Hypothermic persons submerged less than 60 minutes may respond to prolonged resuscitation, but generally only if they can be rewarmed, which may be impractical in the wilderness. If medical help is available rapidly, CPR should be continued until the person has been rewarmed. In hypothermic persons submerged more than 60 minutes, CPR is rarely successful.

What to Look for	What to Do
The person is seen struggling in the water, floating motionless, or lying at the bottom of a body of water.	1. Check the scene. Assess your resources and abilities before attempting a rescue. Rescue of a submerged or drowning person can be dangerous. 2. Rescue the person. Remember, do not become a rescue subject yourself! The following guidelines are suggested for getting a person safely out of the water: reach, throw, row, go: ▪ Reach = Reach with a long object (eg, tree limb or paddle) from shore. ▪ Throw = Throw any object that floats (eg, picnic jug or spare tire) or throw a rope and tow the person to safety.

Continues

What to Look for	What to Do
	■ Row = Use a rowboat, raft, or canoe if available. ■ Go = If trained and skilled, swim to the person. Use a towel or board for them to hold onto. DO NOT let them grab you. This can be a dangerous rescue. **3.** If the person was diving (or it is unknown whether they were diving), suspect a possible spinal injury. Manually stabilize the person while floating on the water's surface. Because most wilderness lakes and rivers contain cold water, consider removing the person from the water the best you can with the resources available. **4.** Check breathing; if absent, start CPR: ■ You need not start CPR if an adult is known to have been submerged more than 60 minutes in warm water. ■ Stop resuscitation after 30 minutes if there are no signs of life, unless the person has been submerged in very cold water. ■ If submersion has been in very cold water, continue resuscitation for at least 60 minutes with concurrent attempts to warm the person. ■ If there is a pulse, continue rescue breathing as long as possible or until breathing resumes. ■ While the person is in the water, give rescue breaths (mouth-to-barrier or mouth-to-mouth). **5.** Evacuate all persons who have been resuscitated. **6.** Persons not requiring CPR and whose only initial symptoms have been coughing or vomiting require close observation but not immediate evacuation; evacuate for medical evaluation if cough or shortness of breath increases.

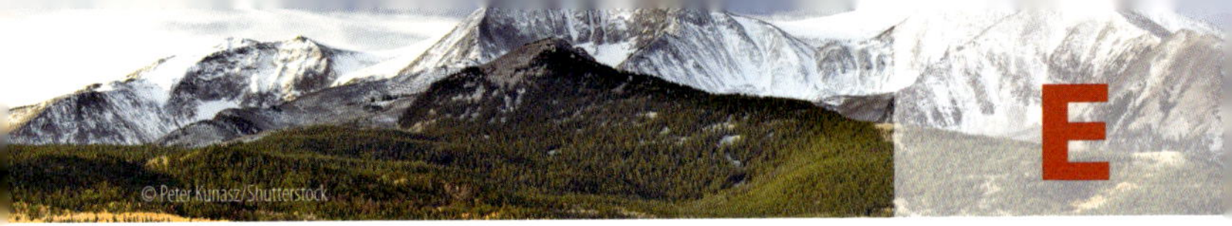

Ear Injuries

Except for disk batteries and live insects, few foreign bodies stuck in a person's ear must be removed immediately. Therefore, evacuate and seek professional medical care for a person with this condition. Attempts to remove a foreign body from the ear can rupture the eardrum or lacerate the ear canal.

What to Look for	What to Do
Object(s) stuck in an ear	1. **DO NOT** use tweezers or try to pry an object out unless the object can be seen near the ear canal opening. 2. Seek professional medical care to remove the object. Except for disk batteries and live insects, few foreign bodies must be removed immediately. 3. For a live insect in the ear canal, shine a small light into the ear. The insect may crawl out toward the light; if it does not, pour warm water into the ear and then drain it. This may drown the insect; regardless of whether it is dead or alive, it should wash out. When draining the water, turn the head to the side. If the insect cannot be removed, seek professional medical care.

Continues

What to Look for	What to Do
Fluids coming from the ear (blood or clear fluid draining from the ear may indicate a skull fracture)	1. **DO NOT** attempt to stop bleeding or clear fluid (cerebrospinal fluid) with or without blood coming from an ear. Doing so could increase pressure on the brain, causing permanent damage. 2. Place a sterile gauze dressing over the ear and loosely bandage it in place to prevent bacteria getting into the brain. 3. Stabilize the head and neck against movement. Tell the person to remain as still as possible. 4. Evacuate and seek professional medical care.

Eye Injuries

DO NOT assume an eye injury is minor. For double vision, pain, or reduced vision, seek medical help. When in doubt, evacuate and seek professional medical help immediately.

What to Look for	What to Do
Blow to the eye, indicated by: ■ A shiner, or black eye, occurring when some of the many delicate blood vessels around the eye rupture ■ Person reports being hit by a fist, ball, or other blunt object	1. Apply ice pack around the eye for 15 minutes. **DO NOT** place ice pack directly on the eye or put pressure on the eye. 2. Have the person keep their eyes closed. 3. Evacuate and seek professional medical care.

What to Look for	What to Do
▪ Broken bone around the eyeball indicated by double vision and the inability to look upward	
Loose object in the eye, indicated by: ▪ Severe pain ▪ Tearing (the body's way of trying to remove the object)	Try, in order, each of the following methods until one is effective: **1.** Have the person blink their eye several times. **2.** Using the eyelashes, gently pull the upper eyelid out and over the lower lid. Have the person blink a few times and let the eye move the object out. **3.** Gently irrigate the eye with clean, warm water. Hold the eyelid open and tell the person to move the eye as it is rinsed. **4.** Examine the lower lid by pulling it down gently. If you see the object, remove it with a moistened gauze pad. **5.** Lift the upper eyelid up and over a cotton swab. If the object is seen, remove it with the corner of a wet gauze pad. **6.** If any of the previously discussed methods are successful, professional medical care is usually not needed unless there is continued pain or itching to the eye.

Continues

What to Look for	What to Do
Cut on the eyeball, indicated by: ■ Cut appearance of the cornea (clear part of the eye) or sclera (white part of the eye) ■ Inner liquid filling of the eye coming out through the wound ■ Cut lid	1. **DO NOT** apply pressure to the eye. 2. Cover both eyes with gauze pads, and lightly wrap a bandage around the head to hold the pads in place. 3. Evacuate and seek professional medical care immediately.
Scratch on eyeball: ■ Symptoms are similar to those of a loose object in the eye. ■ A severe scratch or abrasion may be visible. ■ Person reports changes in vision.	1. Treat as a loose object in the eye. 2. Try sunglasses to soothe the eye. 3. Use pain medication (eg, acetaminophen) according to package directions. A damp cloth over the eyes can provide some relief. 4. If pain persists, patch the eye until symptoms improve. 5. If pain or visual changes last beyond 48 hours, signs of infection develop (such as pus), or a visible ulcer develops on the eye, evacuate and seek professional medical care.
Cut eyelid	1. If only the eyelid is cut, apply a soft, sterile or clean dressing with gentle pressure, and lightly wrap a bandage around the head to hold the pad in place. 2. Evacuate and seek professional medical care for sutures. If not sutured, the eyelid may be permanently droopy or partially closed.

What to Look for	What to Do
Eye avulsion, indicated by: ■ Eye knocked out from its socket	**1.** Cover the eye loosely with a sterile or clean dressing that has been moistened with clean water. Do not try to push the eyeball back into the socket. **2.** Protect the injured eye with a paper cup, a piece of cardboard folded into a cone, or a doughnut-shaped pad made from a roller gauze bandage or a cravat bandage. **3.** Cover the undamaged eye with a patch to stop movement of the damaged eye. **4.** Evacuate and seek professional medical care immediately.
Chemical, smoke, or other irritant in eye	Act immediately: **1.** Hold the eye wide open; flush with warm water for at least 15 minutes or until EMS arrive. If tap water is not available, normal saline or other eye irrigation solution may be used. ■ Irrigate from the nose side of the eye toward the outside to avoid flushing the material into the other eye. ■ Tell the person to roll the eye as much as possible to help wash out the eye. **2.** Loosely bandage the eye or eyes if necessary. **3.** For a chemical eye injury, evacuate and seek professional medical care immediately.

Continues

What to Look for	What to Do
Burns caused by light, indicated by: ■ Person reports looking at a source of ultraviolet light such as sunlight, bright snow, or water ■ Severe pain occurring 1 to 6 hours after exposure	1. Cover both eyes with moist, cool cloths. 2. Give pain medication, if needed. 3. Evacuate and seek professional medical advice.
Hyphema, indicated by: ■ Visible pool of blood in front of the iris of the eye **FIGURE 19**. ■ Impaired vision ■ Pain in eye	1. Keep physical activity to a minimum. 2. Tell the person to keep both eyes closed and cover the affected eye with an eye patch. **DO NOT** apply pressure on the eyeball because further damage can occur. 3. Apply an eye shield (eg, paper or plastic cup) over the eye patch to protect the eye from being struck. 4. Keep the person's head in an elevated and upright position. 5. Evacuate and seek professional medical care immediately.
Penetrating eye injury, indicated by: ■ Object protruding from eye ■ Lid laceration or cut	1. **DO NOT** remove the object. 2. For a long object, place padding around the object to stabilize against movement, and place a paper cup or similar object over the object for protection **FIGURE 20**. 3. For a short object, place a doughnut-shaped pad (formed from a roller gauze bandage or a cravat bandage made from a triangular bandage) around the eye without touching the object, and wrap a bandage around the head to hold the pad in place.

What to Look for	What to Do
	4. Cover both eyes; movement of the uninjured eye will cause movement of the injured eye. **5.** Keep the person flat on their back. **6.** Evacuate and seek professional medical care immediately.
Dry eye, indicated by: ▪ Person complains about an eye being itchy, scratchy, stinging, or tired ▪ Pain and redness ▪ Impaired vision over time	**1.** Have the person blink more often and rest the eyes. **2.** Twice an hour, have the person close their eyes and then move the eyeballs around underneath the closed lids as you count slowly to 10. **3.** **DO NOT** rub the eyes, which can further irritate them. **4.** Apply artificial tears one to two times every hour, which can provide temporary relief. ▪ Liquid drops are fine for mild or intermittent dryness. A gel product lasts longer. Longer lasting than liquid drops or gel are OTC lubricating ointments used every few hours; note that ointments may cause blurry vision so it is best to try them at bedtime.
Conjunctivitis, indicated by: ▪ Redness in the sclera (white part of the eye) ▪ Itching or gritty sensation in the eye ▪ Oozing discharge ▪ Excessive tearing	**If allergic conjunctivitis is suspected:** **1.** Apply cool compresses to the eye. **2.** Apply artificial tears to dilute the offending allergen and relieve some of the itching. Antihistamine drops may also be considered for relieving symptoms but should not be used for more than 2 or 3 days.

Continues

What to Look for	What to Do
■ Swollen eyelids ■ Dried crusts that form during sleep may bind the eyelids together. ■ Discomfort caused by bright lights	**3.** Seek professional medical care if signs and symptoms do not improve after 3 or 4 days of treatment, especially if fever, increased pain, or changes in vision develop. **It is difficult to distinguish between viral and bacterial conjunctivitis. If either is suspected:** **1.** Soak a clean cloth in warm water, wring out the excess water, and apply it to the eye. **2.** Apply artificial tears as needed to provide comfort. **3.** Seek professional medical care for prescription antibiotic eye drops.

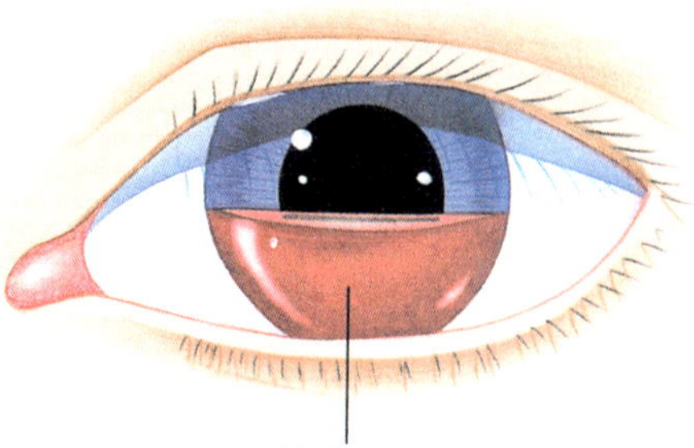

FIGURE 19 Hyphema

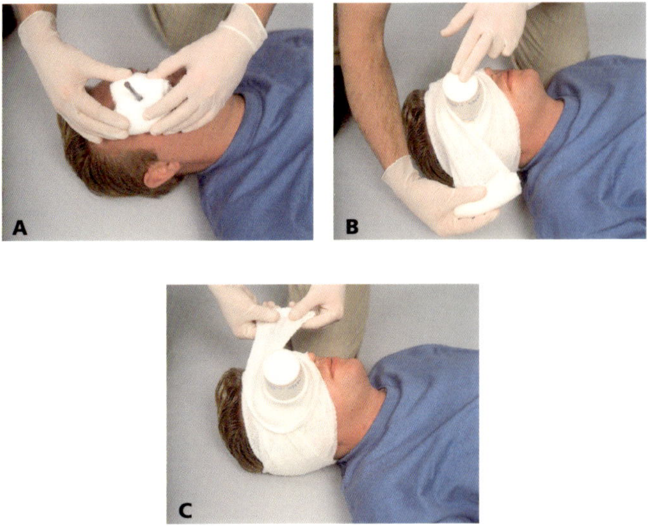

FIGURE 20 Stabilize a long penetrating object against movement. **A**. Place padding around the object. **B**. Place a shield (ie, paper cup or similar object) over, but not touching, the penetrating object to protect the object from being hit. **C**. Cover both eyes to prevent the uninjured eye from moving with the injured eye.

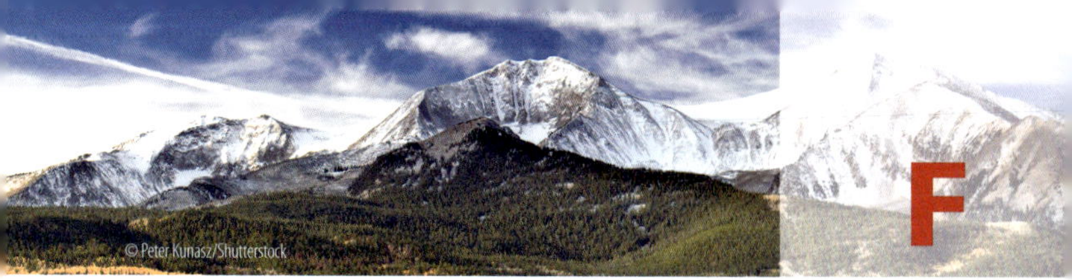

Female Health Problems

Vaginitis

What to Look for	What to Do
■ White or yellowish discharge ■ Pain when urinating ■ Vaginal soreness, burning, and/or itching	1. The woman should wash several times daily with clean water. 2. She should wear loose-fitting underwear and pants. 3. She should wipe from front to back after a bowel movement or after urinating. 4. Seek professional medical help if there is lower abdominal pain and a fever or if foul-smelling vaginal discharge exists.

Urinary Tract Infection

What to Look for	What to Do
■ Frequent urge to urinate ■ Burning sensation while urinating	1. Give fluids—water is best. Avoid caffeine and alcohol. 2. The woman should wear loose-fitting underwear and pants.

What to Look for	What to Do
■ Blood in the urine	**3.** She should wash the area daily. **4.** A hot bath may help relieve pain and itching. **5.** She should wipe from front to back after a bowel movement or after urinating. **6.** Evacuate if symptoms last for 24 hours or if fever and chills occur.

Vaginal Bleeding

For injury-related soft-tissue injuries, use direct pressure to control bleeding. Apply cold to reduce swelling and pain. Apply a diaper-type bandage to hold dressings in place. Never place or pack dressings into the vagina. Evacuate the woman and seek professional medical help.

Noninjury vaginal bleeding can result from various causes, but the care is the same. Have the woman place a sanitary pad over the vaginal opening, and seek professional medical help.

Pregnancy Problems

- The "big three" warning signs of a serious problem are bleeding, abdominal cramps, and weakness. Seek professional medical help ASAP.
- Morning sickness, swollen ankles, and urinary tract infections are not usually dangerous, but seek professional medical advice.
- If a pregnant woman is "spotting," have her lie down on her left side because this improves circulation. Spotting could signal the onset of a miscarriage.

Freezing and Nonfreezing Injuries

Nonfreezing cold injuries such as trench foot can occur when conditions are cold and wet (air temperatures between 32°F and 55°F [0°C and 12.8°C]). Freezing cold injuries such as frostbite and frostnip can occur whenever the air temperature is below freezing (32°F [0°C]).

Frostbite

Frostbite happens only in below-freezing temperatures. It mainly affects the feet, hands, ears, and nose. The most severe consequences of frostbite occur when tissue dies (gangrene) and the affected part might have to be amputated. The longer the tissue stays frozen, the worse the injury. Check for hypothermia in any frostbitten person.

What to Look for	What to Do

Before thawing, frostbite can be classified as superficial or deep:
■ Superficial frostbite:
  ■ Skin is white, red, purple, gray, yellow, or waxy.
  ■ The affected part feels very cold and numb. There might be tingling, stinging, or an aching sensation.
	1. Get the person out of the cold and to a warm place. If possible, do not let the person use a frozen extremity until professional medical care is reached.
	2. Remove any wet clothing and constricting items, such as rings, that could impair blood circulation.
	3. **DO NOT** attempt to thaw the part if:
	  ■ Medical care is less than 2 hours away.
	  ■ The affected area has thawed.
	  ■ Shelter, warm water, and a container are not available.
	  ■ Risk of refreezing exists.

What to Look for	What to Do
▪ The skin surface feels stiff or crusty and the underlying tissue feels soft when depressed gently and firmly. ▪ Deep frostbite: ▪ The affected part feels cold, hard, and solid and cannot be depressed; it feels like a piece of wood or frozen meat. ▪ Skin in the affected body part is pale or black and waxy. ▪ A painfully cold part suddenly stops hurting.	**4.** Use the wet, rapid rewarming method if: ▪ Medical care is more than 2 hours away. ▪ There exists no further risk of refreezing of the affected area. ▪ Shelter, warm water, and a container are available. Although wet, rapid rewarming is recommended, you may be unable to avoid slow thawing; you should allow slow thawing if it is the only method available. **5.** Wet, *rapid rewarming method*: Place the frostbitten part in warm water (100°F to 104°F [38°C to 40°C]). **DO NOT** use other heat sources (eg, fire, space heater, oven). If you do not have a thermometer, you can put your hand into the water for 30 seconds to test that it is warm but not hot enough to burn. Maintain the water temperature by adding warm water as needed. Rewarming usually takes 20 to 40 minutes or until the part becomes soft and pliable to touch. Air dry the area; **DO NOT** rub. To help control the severe pain during rewarming, give the person ibuprofen as directed on the label. For ear or facial injuries, it is best to apply warm, moist cloths, changing them frequently. *Cautions:* ▪ **DO NOT** use water hotter than 104°F (40°C): burns can result. ▪ **DO NOT** use water cooler than 98°F (37°C): it will not thaw frostbite rapidly enough. ▪ **DO NOT** break any blisters.

Continues

What to Look for	What to Do
	■ **DO NOT** rub or massage the affected part—ice crystals can be pushed into body cells, rupturing them. ■ **DO NOT** rub the affected part with ice or snow. ■ **DO NOT** rewarm the part with a heating pad, hot-water bottle, stove, sunlamp, radiator, or exhaust pipe or over a fire. Excessive temperatures cannot be controlled, and burns can result. ■ **DO NOT** allow the person to drink alcoholic beverages. Alcohol dilates blood vessels and causes loss of body heat. ■ **DO NOT** allow the person to smoke. Smoking constricts blood vessels, thus impairing circulation. ■ **DO NOT** rewarm if there is any possibility of refreezing. ■ **DO NOT** allow the thawed part to refreeze because the ice crystals formed will be larger and more damaging. If refreezing is likely or even possible, it is better to leave the affected part frozen. ■ **DO NOT** use the dry rewarming technique (putting the person's hands in your armpits) for frostbite. The dry rewarming technique takes three to four times longer than the wet, rapid method to thaw frozen tissue. Slow rewarming results in greater tissue damage than rapid rewarming. ■ **DO NOT** rewarm if close to a medical facility.

What to Look for	What to Do

After thawing, frostbite can be categorized by degrees, similar to the classification of burns:
■ First-degree frostbite
  ■ The affected part is warm, swollen, and tender.
■ Second-degree frostbite
  ■ Blisters form within minutes to hours after thawing and enlarge over several days.
■ Third-degree frostbite
  ■ Blisters are small and contain red-blue or purple fluid. The surrounding skin may be red or blue and might not blanch when pressure is applied.
	After thawing:
	1. If the feet are affected, do not allow the person to walk. The feet will be impossible to use after they are rewarmed unless only the toes are affected.
	2. Protect the affected area from contact with clothing and bedding.
	3. Place bulky, dry, clean gauze on the affected part and between the toes and the fingers to absorb moisture and keep them from sticking together.
	4. Slightly elevate the affected part above heart level to reduce pain and swelling.
	5. Apply aloe vera gel to promote skin healing.
	6. Give ibuprofen according to package directions to limit pain and inflammation.
	7. Give fluids if the person is alert and can swallow.
	8. Protect against refreezing.
	9. Evacuate and seek professional medical care as soon as possible.

Frostnip

Frostnip is caused when parts of the skin are chilled but not frozen. Frostnip should be taken seriously because it could be the first sign of impending frostbite. It may be difficult to tell the difference between frostnip and frostbite.

What to Look for	What to Do
Signs of frostnip, indicated by: ■ Yellow to gray skin color ■ Frost (ice crystals) on the skin ■ Initial tingling or numbness that may become painful	**1.** Get the person out of the cold and to a warm place. **2.** Gently warm the affected area by placing it against a warm body part (eg, have the person put their bare hands under their armpits) or by applying a warm chemical heat pack covered by a cloth. For the nose, breathe with cupped hands over the nose. **3.** **DO NOT** rub the area.

Trench Foot/Immersion Foot

Immersion foot, also known as trench foot, occurs in nonfreezing cold and wet conditions when the skin on the feet is exposed to moisture and cold for prolonged periods. This takes several days to occur.

What to Look for	What to Do
■ Itching, numbness, or tingling pain in the feet ■ Swollen feet ■ Pale, ashen, or gray skin that feels cold when touched ■ Wrinkled skin over the soles of the feet ■ Red, blue, or gray splotches on the skin, sometimes with open weeping or bleeding	**1.** Dry the skin. **2.** Rewarm the foot gradually. **3.** Care for open weeping areas by cleansing with mild soap and water and applying breathable dressings. **4.** Evacuate.

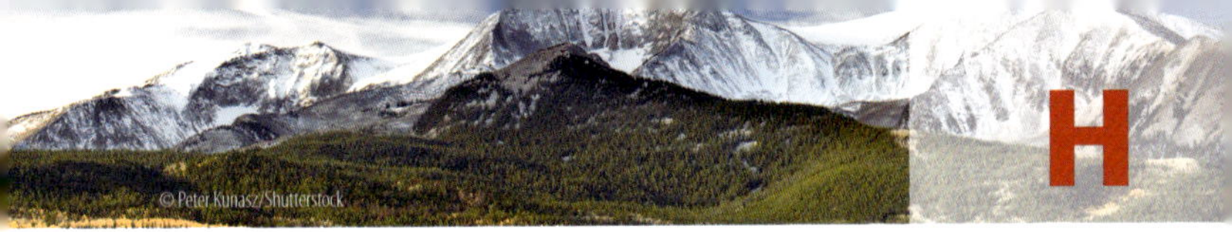

Head Injuries

Head injuries include any damage to the scalp, skull, or brain. Spinal injuries (eg, neck and back injuries) can also be present in people with a head injury. Stabilize against movement until you have obtained additional evidence that an injury to the spinal cord is not likely (see the section on *Spinal Injury*).

Scalp Wound

What to Look for	What to Do
Scalp wound	**1.** Control bleeding by pressing on the wound. Replace any skin flap to its original position and apply pressure. Another option is applying an ice pack or instant cold pack to control bleeding. **2.** If you suspect a skull fracture, **DO NOT** apply excessive pressure; doing so may push bone pieces into the brain. Press on the edges of the wound to help control bleeding. **3.** Apply a dry, sterile, or clean dressing. **4.** Keep the head and shoulders raised if no spinal injury is suspected. **5.** If bleeding continues, remove the first blood-soaked dressing and apply well-aimed direct pressure with a new dressing.

Continues

What to Look for	What to Do
	6. Evacuate immediately if any of the following occurs: ■ The wound is extensive. ■ There is significant facial damage. ■ Signs of concussion occur (eg, nausea and vomiting, headache, drowsiness).

Skull Fracture

What to Look for	What to Do
■ Pain ■ Skull deformity ■ Bleeding from an ear or the nose ■ Leakage of clear, watery fluid from an ear or the nose (cerebrospinal fluid) ■ Discoloration around the eyes or behind ears appearing several hours after the injury ■ Unequal-size pupils of the eye ■ Heavy scalp bleeding (skull and/or brain tissue may be exposed) ■ Penetrating or impaled object	**1.** Cover wounds with a sterile dressing. **2.** Control bleeding by pressing the edges of the wound and gently on the center of it to avoid pressing bone pieces into the brain. A doughnut-shaped pad is useful in applying pressure around the edges of a suspected skull fracture. **3.** Stabilize the neck against movement unless you have obtained additional evidence that an injury to the spinal cord is not likely. (see the section on *Spinal Injury*). **4.** Evacuate immediately. **5.** *Cautions:* **DO NOT** clean the wound. **DO NOT** remove an embedded object. **DO NOT** stop blood or clear fluid that is draining from an ear or the nose. **DO NOT** press on the fractured area. **DO NOT** move the head, neck, or spine.

Brain Injury (Concussion)

A concussion is a type of traumatic brain injury (TBI) caused by a bump, blow, or jolt to the head that can change the way the brain normally works.

Most concussions (80% to 90%) resolve within 7 to 10 days, but some people take much longer to recover.

What to Look for	What to Do
Signs of concussion or mild traumatic brain injury, which may worsen over minutes or hours: *Thinking/remembering symptoms:* ▪ Difficulty thinking clearly ▪ Feeling slowed down ▪ Difficulty concentrating ▪ Difficulty remembering new information *Physical symptoms:* ▪ Headache ▪ Fuzzy or blurred vision ▪ Nausea or vomiting (early on) ▪ Dizziness ▪ Sensitivity to noise or light ▪ Balance problems ▪ Feeling tired, having no energy	**1.** If unresponsive, do a Primary Assessment (see *Finding Out What Is Wrong* section). **2.** If a neck injury exists or if the person is unresponsive: **a.** **DO NOT** move the head, neck, or spine. **b.** Tell the person to remain as still as possible. **3.** Evacuate immediately if the person: ▪ Looks very drowsy or cannot be awakened. ▪ Has one pupil (the black part in the middle of the eye) that is larger than the other. ▪ Has a seizure. ▪ Cannot recognize people or places. ▪ Becomes more and more confused, restless, or agitated. ▪ Exhibits unusual behavior. ▪ Develops an altered mental status or becomes unresponsive (VPU on the AVPU scale). ▪ Has a headache that gets worse and/or does not go away. ▪ Has repeated vomiting or nausea. ▪ Has slurred speech.

Continues

What to Look for	What to Do
Emotional/mood symptoms: ■ Irritability ■ Sadness ■ More emotional ■ Nervousness or anxiety *Sleep disturbance symptoms:* ■ Sleeping more than usual ■ Sleeping less than usual ■ Trouble falling asleep	**4.** Following the injury, the person should: ■ Get plenty of sleep at night and rest during the day. ■ Avoid visual and sensory stimuli, including video games and loud music. ■ Ease into normal activities slowly, not all at once. ■ Avoid strenuous physical activities that increase the heart rate or require a lot of concentration. ■ Avoid driving, cycling, operating machinery, or playing sports until assessed by a health care provider. ■ Avoid anything that could cause another blow to the head or body. ■ **DO NOT** use aspirin or anti-inflammatory medications such as ibuprofen or naproxen due to the risk of bleeding. Acetaminophen (Tylenol) can be used for postconcussion headaches.

Heart Attack

In a heart attack, the heart muscle tissue dies because its blood supply has been severely reduced or stopped.

What to Look for	What to Do
Although sometimes difficult to determine, symptoms of a heart attack can include: ■ Chest discomfort that feels like pressure, squeezing, or fullness, usually in the center of the chest. It may also be felt in the jaw, shoulder, arms, or back. It may last for more than 5 minutes, or it may come and go.	**1.** Have the person sit, with knees raised, and lean against a stable support (eg, wall, fence post, tree trunk). Try to keep the person calm. **DO NOT** allow the person to walk. Doing so can put more stress on the heart.

What to Look for	What to Do
■ Sweating or "cold sweats" ■ Light-headedness or dizziness ■ Nausea or vomiting ■ Numbness, aching, or tingling in the arm (usually the left arm) ■ Shortness of breath ■ Weakness or fatigue, especially in older adults Women and older adults experience the typical signs and symptoms of a heart attack. However, women and older adults are more likely than men to have milder signs and symptoms of a heart attack that can extend over many hours, days, or weeks leading up to the heart attack, such as: ■ Shortness of breath ■ Nausea or vomiting ■ An ache in the chest ■ Sore jaw ■ Strange feeling in arm ■ Upper back pain ■ Flulike symptoms ■ Dizziness	**2.** Loosen any tight clothing. **3.** Ask if the person takes any chest pain medication, such as nitroglycerin, for a known heart condition, and help them take it. **4.** If the person is alert, able to swallow, and not allergic to aspirin, help the victim take one aspirin (325 mg) or two to four low-dose aspirins (81 mg each). For faster results, have the person chew the aspirin before swallowing. **5.** Monitor breathing. If the person becomes unresponsive and stops breathing, begin CPR (see Cardiac Arrest section for CPR). If they are unresponsive and are breathing, place them on their side (recovery position). **6.** Evacuate and seek professional medical care immediately.

Heat-Related Illnesses

Heat illnesses include a range of disorders. Some are common, but only heatstroke is life threatening. Untreated heatstroke may result in death.

Heatstroke

Two Types of Heatstroke

There are two types of heatstroke: *classic* and *exertional* TABLE 1.

TABLE 1 Classic or Exertional Heatstroke?

Characteristics	Classic	Exertional
Age group usually affected	Older people	Men, 15–45 years
Claims many people at the same time	During heat waves	During athletic competition
Health status of people	Chronically ill	Healthy and physically fit
Activity at the time of the incident	Sedentary	Strenuous exercise
Medication use	Common	Usually none
Sweating	Absent	Often present (50% of people)

What to Look for	What to Do
▪ Extremely hot skin ▪ Skin that is usually dry, but may be wet from sweating related to strenuous work or exercise ▪ Altered mental status ranging from slight confusion, agitation, and disorientation to possible seizures or unresponsiveness ▪ Flushed skin ▪ Flulike symptoms (headache, body aches, nausea, and sometimes vomiting) ▪ Body temperature, usually above 104°F (40°C) causing a feeling of burning up	**1.** Move the person from the hot environment to a cooler, shaded place. **2.** Evacuate and seek professional medical care immediately. **3.** A person who cannot be taken to a medical facility quickly should be cooled by any means possible. The order of effective cooling is: ▪ **Whole-body cold-water immersion.** First, remove clothing down to the person's underwear and then: ▪ Submerge the person's body and extremities up to the neck in a bath of cold water or tub of ice water. The colder the water, the faster the rate of cooling. OR ▪ Have the person sit or lay down on a plastic sheet or tarp. Hold the sides up and apply water and crushed ice. Keep the sides upright to keep the mixture in place and move the tarp to keep the water moving around the person.

Continues

What to Look for	What to Do
	OR ■ Use a natural body of water (eg, stream, pond, river, or lake) to submerge a person and help cool them off. **DO NOT** leave someone suffering from heatstroke in a body of water alone. ■ **Spray or douse cold water** repeatedly on the person's skin and fan them vigorously. This method is half as fast as immersion cooling. ■ **Ice packs.** Ice packs should cover the entire body. If chemical cold packs are used, they should be applied to the cheeks, palms, and soles rather than the skin covering the neck, armpits, and groin. Ice packs have greater cooling capacity than chemical cold packs. **4.** Stop cooling when the person's mental status improves, when the person's body temperature moves back into the normal range, or after 20 minutes, or when EMS arrives. **5.** **DO NOT** give the person ibuprofen or aspirin. While helpful in cases of high body temperatures caused by infectious diseases, they are not effective in heat-related illnesses.

Heat Exhaustion

What to Look for	What to Do
▪ Clammy or sweaty skin, but not hot skin. ▪ Severe thirst ▪ Fatigue ▪ Dizzy ▪ Flu like symptoms (headache, body aches, and nausea) ▪ Shortness of breath ▪ Rapid heart rate Heat exhaustion differs from heatstroke because the affected person has (1) skin that is clammy but not hot, (2) no altered mental status, and (3), no elevated body temperature.	Suspect heat exhaustion: Uncontrolled heat exhaustion can evolve into heatstroke. **1.** Move the person to a cool, shaded area. **2.** Have the person remove excess clothing. **3.** If the person can swallow, give lightly salted cool water (dissolve ¼ teaspoon salt in 1 quart of water), a commercial sports drink, or fruit juice. If none of these options are available, give the person cold water. **DO NOT** give salt tablets. **4.** Cool the person, but not as aggressively as for heatstroke. **5.** If no improvement is seen within 30 minutes, evacuate. Recovery may take up to 24 hours.

Hyponatremia (Water Intoxication)

When sodium is flushed out of the body by drinking too much water, hyponatremia, nicknamed "water intoxication," can occur. Sodium loss is seldom a problem unless the person sweats profusely for long periods and drinks large quantities of water.

What to Look for

- Person reports drinking too much water (>1 quart [about 1 L] per hour)
- Vomiting clear fluid
- Profuse sweating for long periods
- Frequent urination (clear urine)
- Dizziness, weakness, nausea, headache
- Altered mental status
- Severe sodium loss may result in seizures or unresponsiveness and can be fatal.

What to Do

1. Move the person to a cool location.
2. **DO NOT** give more fluids.
3. Give salty foods. **DO NOT** give salt tablets because they can irritate the stomach and cause nausea and vomiting.
4. Evacuate for:
   - No improvement
   - Altered mental status
   - Seizure
   - Vomiting
   - Shortness of breath
   - Collapse

Heat Cramps

What to Look for

- Painful spasms in abdominal muscles or extremities
- Heavy sweating

What to Do

Relief may take several hours.

1. Have the person rest in a cool place.
2. Give lightly salted cool water (dissolve a quarter teaspoon [1.25 mL] of salt in 1 quart [about 1 L] of water) or a commercial sports drink. **DO NOT** give salt tablets.
3. Lightly stretch and massage the cramped muscles.
4. Apply an ice pack to the cramped muscles.

Heat Syncope

What to Look for	What to Do
Signs of heat syncope occur immediately after strenuous activity in a hot environment. ■ Dizziness ■ Fainting	**1.** If the person is unresponsive, check their breathing. The person usually recovers quickly. **2.** If the person fell, check for injuries. **3.** Have the person rest and lie down in a cool area. **4.** Wet the skin with a cool, damp cloth or by splashing water on the face. **5.** If the person is not nauseated and is alert and able to swallow, give lightly salted cool water (dissolve a quarter teaspoon [1.25 mL] of salt in 1 quart [about 1 L] of water) or a commercial sports drink. **DO NOT** give salt tablets.

Heat Edema

What to Look for	What to Do
■ Swollen ankles and feet ■ Occurs during first few days in a hot environment.	**1.** Have the person wear support stockings. **2.** Elevate the person's legs.

Heat Rash (Prickly Heat)

What to Look for	What to Do
■ Itchy rash on skin wet from sweating ■ Seen in humid regions after prolonged sweating	**1.** Dry and cool the person's skin. **2.** Limit heat exposure.

Hypothermia

Cold Stress

Cold stress develops when a person has been exposed to a cold environment. They may be shivering but will be alert and can move and care for themselves. Many people in the outdoors can mistake being cold as being hypothermic. **DO NOT** mistake cold stress for hypothermia. If not paying attention, a cold-stressed person can become hypothermic.

What to Look for	What to Do
A person has been exposed to a cold environment and has these signs: ■ Alert and shivering ■ Can move and care for themselves	Suspect cold stress, but not hypothermia. **1.** Allow the person to remove their own wet clothing and to put on dry clothing. **2.** Give high-calorie food or drink. **3.** Move around; exercise to warm up. **4.** Consider using a warm shower or bath.

Hypothermia

Hypothermia happens when the body's temperature (98.6°F [37°C]) drops more than 2°. Hypothermia does not require subfreezing temperatures. Severe hypothermia is life threatening. Check for possible frostbite.

What to Look for	What to Do
Any of the signs of mild, moderate, or severe hypothermia	Take the following actions for all people with suspected hypothermia: 1. Get the person out of the cold. Treat hypothermia before treating frostbite. 2. Handle the person gently. 3. Replace wet clothing with dry clothing only when the person is inside or has other protection from the cold. 4. Add insulation (eg, extra clothing, blankets, towels, pillows, sleeping bag) beneath and around the person. Cover the person's head (eg, stocking cap, hood). 5. Cover the person with a vapor barrier (eg, tarp, trash bags with a hole cut out for the face) to prevent heat loss. **DO NOT** cover the mouth or nose. If the person's clothing is dry or damp, leave it on if you know that EMS will arrive in less than 30 minutes. If the clothing is very wet, there is shelter, and EMS is more than 30 minutes away, remove the wet clothing. If unable to remove wet clothing, place the vapor barrier between clothing and insulation. For a dry person, the vapor barrier can be placed outside the insulation. Ideally, using two vapor barriers (one against the person and one outside the insulating layer) offers more protection.

Continues

What to Look for	What to Do
Signs of mild hypothermia: ■ Vigorous, uncontrollable shivering ■ Awake and alert ■ Complains of feeling cold—painful hands and feet ■ Can answer questions intelligently	**1.** If in a warm dry shelter, have the person sit or lie down for at least 30 minutes. **2.** Warm the arms up to the elbows, and the lower legs up to the knees, in 104°F to 113°F (40°C to 45°C) water. **3.** Add insulation (eg, extra clothing, blankets, towels, pillows, sleeping bag) beneath and around the person. Cover the person's head (eg, hat, hood). **4.** Give high-calorie (sugary) nonalcoholic and noncaffeinated food or drinks to maintain shivering. Shivering rewarms a person who is cold-stressed or mildly hypothermic.
■ The "umbles" beginning to appear: ■ Grumbles ■ Mumbles ■ Fumbles ■ Stumbles ■ Tumbles	**5.** Apply heat to the chest, armpits, and back (in this order). Upper torso rewarming is more effective than extremity rewarming. Use large electric pads, electric blankets, or warm water bottles. Place thin insulation between the skin and heat source to prevent burning the skin. Check the skin every 20 to 30 minutes for signs of burning. **6.** **DO NOT** use warm showers or baths for rewarming. This method may be considered for persons who are cold stressed, but not for even a mildly hypothermic person. It causes too many medical complications.

What to Look for	What to Do
	7. **DO NOT** use small chemical heat packs for rewarming. These packs (eg, used for hand and foot warming) do not provide sufficient heat to affect the core body temperature. They can cause burns. 8. Use the body-to-body method for a mild hypothermic person when there will be a long delay in getting professional medical care. In such a case, the person must be warmed by any available external heat source. 9. Monitor the person for at least 30 minutes. 10. Evacuate to a medical facility if no improvement.
Signs of moderate hypothermia: ■ Shivering stops ■ The "umbles" worsen ■ Does not want to move much; may be sleepy ■ Confused and indifferent to surroundings ■ Skin that is pale or blue and cold when touched	1. Evacuate immediately. 2. Handle gently. 3. Keep the person flat (horizontal). **DO NOT** raise the legs. 4. **DO NOT** allow standing or walking. 5. **DO NOT** massage the person's body. 6. **DO NOT** give any drink or food. 7. Insulate and apply a vapor barrier. 8. Apply heat to the chest, armpits, and back (in that order). Upper torso rewarming is more effective than extremity rewarming. Use large electric pads, electric blankets, or warm water bottles. Place thin insulation between the skin and heat source to prevent burning the skin. Check the skin every 20 to 30 minutes for signs of burning.

Continues

What to Look for	What to Do
Signs of severe hypothermia: ■ Barely responsive or unresponsive ■ Rigid and stiff muscles ■ Skin that feels ice cold and appears blue ■ Slow, shallow, or absent breathing and a weak, slow, or absent pulse (heartbeat) ■ Appears dead. The signs of life—heartbeat (pulse) and breathing—may be very difficult to detect.	**1.** Evacuate immediately. **2.** Treat as moderate hypothermia. **3.** Provide resuscitation if needed. Feel for a pulse at the carotid artery (next to the hard lump [larynx] at the front of the throat) for 1 minute. If no pulse is felt after 1 minute, begin CPR. An AED can be used. **4.** **DO NOT** start CPR if the person: ■ Has been submerged in cold water for more than 1 hour. ■ Has obvious fatal injuries. ■ Is frozen (eg, ice in mouth and throat). ■ Has a chest that is stiff and cannot be compressed.

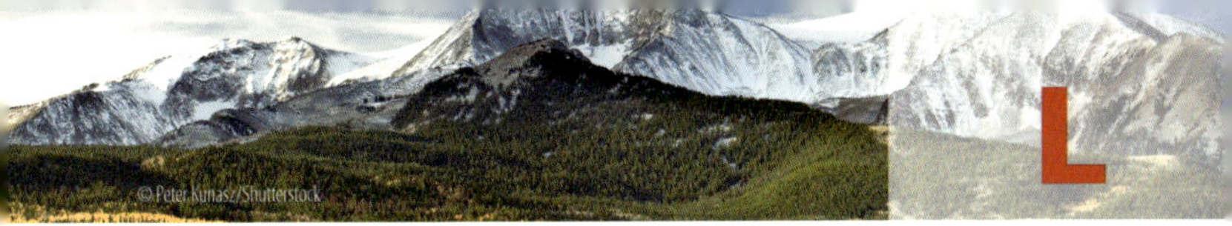
© Peter Kunasz/Shutterstock

Lightning Injuries

Lightning is an electrical discharge associated with thunderstorms. The "Rule of 70s" for lightning strikes indicates that 70% occur in the afternoons, 70% occur during the summer months, 70% of persons survive but may be injured or burned, 70% of persons have an aftereffect such as a hearing/visual/neurological impairment, and 70% of strikes involve only one person. Lightning kills by stopping the heart and breathing.

What to Look for

- No breathing
- Seizures, paralysis, and unresponsive (results if the central nervous system is damaged)
- Minor burns. Most people believe that a person struck by lightning will be severely burned. However, owing to the flashover effect, most people have only the following types of minor burns:
  - *Punctate burns* (small, circular injuries resembling cigarette burns)
  - *Feathering or ferning burns* (injuries often resembling feather- fern-, or vine-like patterns)
  - *Linear burns* (injuries appearing as relatively straight lines)
  - Burns from ignited clothing and heated metal

What to Do

1. If more than one person has been struck by lightning at the same time, go to the quiet and motionless person first, check for breathing and, if absent, begin CPR.
2. If the person is unresponsive but breathing, place the person on their side.
3. Because spinal injuries can occur with lightning strikes, precautions should be taken to stabilize the spine.
4. Check for and treat injuries (fractures, dislocations, burns).
5. Evacuate all people struck.

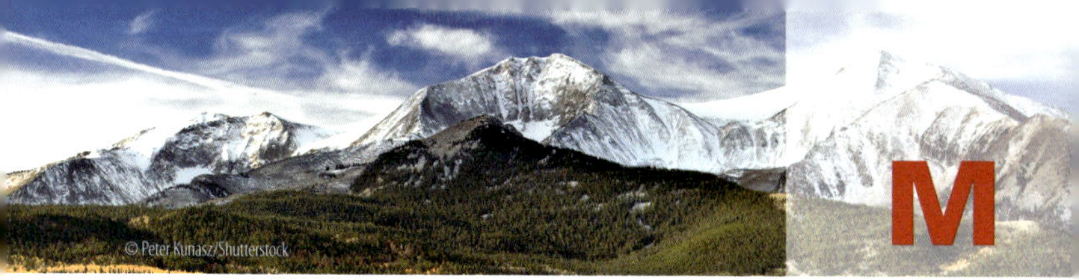

Marine Animal Injuries

What to Look for	What to Do
Bite, rip, or puncture: ▪ Sharks ▪ Barracudas ▪ Eels ▪ Seals	**1.** Monitor breathing. **2.** Control bleeding. **3.** Wash wound with soap and water. **4.** Flush the area with water under pressure (eg, from a faucet or water bottle). **5.** Treat for shock.
Sting: ▪ Jellyfish ▪ Portuguese man-of-war ▪ Sea anemone ▪ Fire coral	**1.** If you have full-strength vinegar (5% acetic acid), spray or pour it over the area for at least 30 seconds. Controversy exists about using vinegar. **2.** Using tweezers or gloved hands, gently but quickly remove tentacles attached to the skin. **DO NOT** scrape, shave, or rub the tentacles off. **3.** Soak the affected skin in nonscalding hot water, in a hot shower, or apply a heat pack for 20–45 minutes. This step can be repeated for pain control.

What to Look for	What to Do
	4. To reduce pain, consider applying over-the-counter lidocaine or benzocaine spray. After applying, **DO NOT** apply hot water again to avoid burns. **5.** **DO NOT** use the following unproven remedies: human urine, meat tenderizer, alcohol, baking soda, compression bandage, or ice pack. **6.** Monitor the person for an allergic reaction and absent breathing.
Venomous bite: ■ Sea snake ■ Octopus ■ Cone snail	**1.** Monitor breathing. **2.** Control bleeding. **3.** Apply pressure bandage on entire arm or leg.
Puncture (by spine): ■ Stingray ■ Scorpion fish ■ Stonefish ■ Starfish ■ Catfish	**1.** Soak the area in hot water for 30 to 90 minutes or until the pain subsides. **DO NOT** use water that is hot enough to burn. **2.** Remove pieces of debris with tweezers. **3.** Wash the area with soap and water. **4.** Flush the area with water under pressure. **5.** Treat the wound.

Motion Sickness

What to Look for	What to Do
Occurs while traveling by car, truck, van, bus, train, ship, or airplane ■ Sweating ■ Dizziness ■ Pale skin ■ Nausea, sometimes leading to vomiting ■ Headache ■ Fatigue	**1.** If the person is susceptible to motion sickness, they should sit near the midsection of a plane, boat, bus, train, or car. People susceptible to motion sickness should not read; should look far ahead to the horizon, not to the sides; and should avoid overeating. **2.** A person susceptible to motion sickness should try taking dimenhydrinate (Dramamine) or a physician-prescribed scopolamine patch 1 hour before traveling (follow label directions). **3.** Stop activity if possible. **4.** Give over-the-counter antinausea pills (such as Dramamine or Bonine). **5.** Give ginger, either as a solid or liquid, or in capsules taken on an empty stomach. **6.** Use thumb pressure or an acupressure wristband (Sea-Band or Psi Band) to apply pressure in the center of the inner wrist between the two forearm bones, two finger widths from the wrist crease. Press three to five times firmly for 1 minute, and then repeat on the other arm.

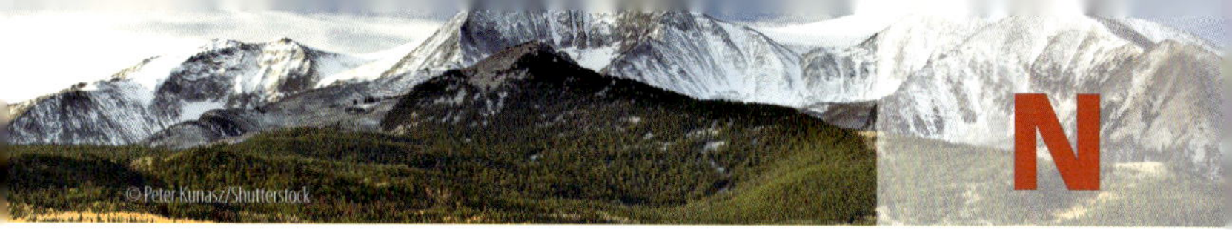

Nose Injuries

What to Look for	What to Do
Broken nose, indicated by: ▪ Pain, swelling, and a possible crooked appearance ▪ Bleeding and difficulty breathing through nostrils ▪ Black eyes appearing 1 to 2 days after injury	**1.** If bleeding, care for the nosebleed. **2.** Encourage the person to spit out the blood as opposed to swallowing it. **3.** Apply an ice pack for 15 minutes. **4.** Medical help can be delayed. **5.** **DO NOT** try to straighten a crooked nose.
Nosebleed	**1.** If nose was hit, suspect a broken nose. **2.** Have the person sit leaning slightly forward. **3.** Pinch nostrils together for 10 minutes. **4.** If bleeding has not stopped, have the person gently blow or sniff their nose to get rid of ineffective blood clots. Pinch nostrils together again for 10 minutes. **5.** If bleeding continues, try other methods in addition to nose pinching, such as applying an ice pack, applying light pressure to the upper lip, or spraying decongestant spray in nostrils. **6.** Medical help is not usually needed. If bleeding continues, evacuate.

Continues

What to Look for	What to Do
Foreign object (a problem mainly with children)	Try one or more of these methods to remove an object: ■ Have the person gently blow their nose while compressing the opposite nostril.
	■ If an object is visible, pull the object out with tweezers. **DO NOT** push the object deeper. ■ Induce sneezing by sniffing pepper. ■ Evacuate if the object cannot be removed.

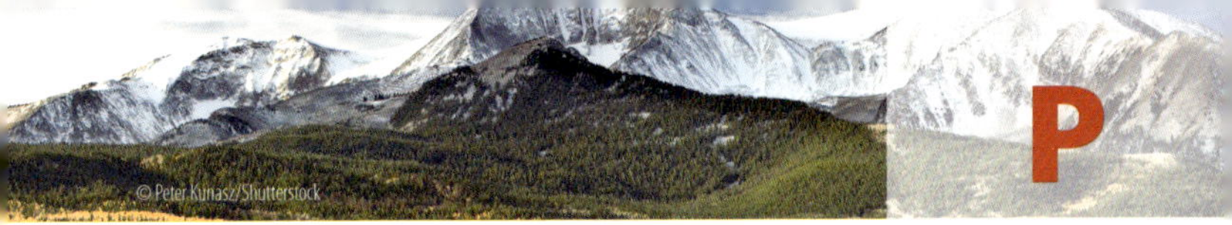

Plant-Related Problems

Plant-Induced Dermatitis: Poison Ivy, Poison Oak, and Poison Sumac

Poison ivy can be found in every state, except Hawaii and Alaska. Poison oak grows in some eastern states and along the West Coast. Poison sumac is found mainly in swampy areas on the East Coast, especially in the Southeast.

Poison ivy growing in one area may not look anything like poison ivy found halfway across the country, and poison oak of the East is very different from poison oak in the West. However, the dermatitis these plants cause, and the treatment, is similar **FIGURE 21**.

About 50% of the people exposed to these plants break out in a rash. The "poison" in these plants is the chemical urushiol, which is found in the sap. All parts of the plant—leaves, stems, roots, flowers, and berries—contain urushiol oil.

An allergic reaction may begin as early as 6 hours after exposure with a line of small blisters where the skin brushed against the plant, followed by redness, swelling, and larger blisters. The blister fluid does not contain the irritant. Usually, the onset of symptoms is 24 to 72 hours after exposure.

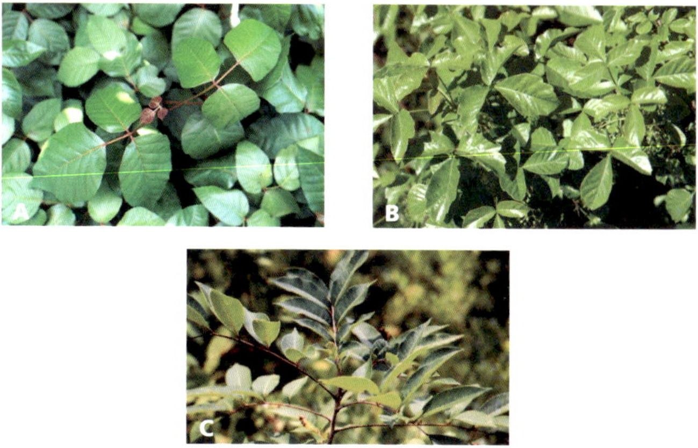

FIGURE 21 Remember that poisonous plants growing in one area may not look anything like the same plant found across the country. **A.** Poison ivy. **B.** Poison oak. **C.** Poison sumac.

As long as 2 weeks after the initial eruption, the rash may appear on other areas of the body. This can be explained by either (1) skin that was exposed to less urushiol or (2) that different parts of the body absorb and react differently to urushiol.

Poison ivy, oak, and sumac dermatitis are self-limiting conditions. Without any treatment, a mild case of any of these will often disappear in about 2 weeks. Usually the discomfort is significant, and the first aid procedures discussed here do not cure the condition but simply ease the suffering.

Over-the-counter (OTC) hydrocortisone cream or ointment (1%) offers little benefit. Seek professional medical advice for severe cases.

Do not worry about spreading the rash to others; it is not contagious. However, animals can carry the oil on their fur and smoke from burning plants can carry particles of the oil. Both can affect an allergic person.

What to Look for	What to Do
Known contact within 5 minutes for people with sensitive skin and up to 1 hour for people with moderately sensitive skin	**1.** Move away from any smoke or fire and gently wipe skin with rubbing alcohol. **DO NOT** rub it in. **2.** Next, or if rubbing alcohol is not available, wash the skin with lots of cold running water. Soap is not necessary, but if used, rinse with lots of cold running water. **DO NOT** scrub the skin. **3.** **DO NOT** use gasoline.
Mild dermatitis: itching	**1.** Apply any of the following: ▪ Colloidal oatmeal bath (Aveeno Soothing Bath Treatments) ▪ Baking soda paste (1 teaspoon water mixed with 3 teaspoons baking soda) ▪ Calamine lotion ▪ Aluminum acetate solution (Burow's solution) ▪ Urushiol solvent product (Zanfel or Tecnu) ▪ Physician-prescribed medication **2.** If none of these are available, the application of an OTC hydrocortisone may be beneficial.
Moderate dermatitis: itching and swelling	**1.** Treat the same as for mild signs and symptoms **2.** Apply a physician-prescribed steroid ointment

Continues

What to Look for	What to Do
Severe dermatitis: itching, swelling, and blisters	**1.** Treat the same as for mild and moderate symptoms. **2.** Apply a physician-prescribed topical or oral steroid. **3.** Evacuate and seek professional medical care if the person inhales smoke from a burning plant or if the reaction involves the face, eyes, genitals, or large areas of the body.

Cactus Spines

Cacti grow in hot, sunny, dry environments. They grow in many sizes and shapes and are usually covered in spines or needles. When the skin is pricked, it causes pain and redness. If not removed, the skin can become inflamed and infected.

What to Look for	What to Do
Medium or large spine(s) embedded in the skin	**1.** Remove with tweezers or pliers by: **a.** Grasping the spine close to the skin. **b.** Slowly pulling the spine out in the same direction that the spine entered. **2.** Clean and treat the small wound with antibiotic ointment and dressing.

What to Look for	What to Do
Hairlike small needles (numbering in the dozens to hundreds) embedded in the skin	**1.** Use any of the following methods. When combined, methods a and b below are considered to be the most effective method for removing most of the needles. No matter which method you choose, **DO NOT** allow the person to suck needles out because they can lodge in the tongue, gums, or throat. **a.** Remove as many needles as you can with tweezers. A magnifying glass may help locate the needles. This method will not remove all small needles. **b.** Use glue. Spread a thin layer of white wood-working glue (ie, Elmer's Glue-All) or rubber cement onto the affected area. **DO NOT** use Super Glue. Press gauze over the glue and wait for it to dry (30 minutes). Gently roll or pull the gauze up from the skin. **c.** Try using duct tape (may remove up to 30% of the needles even after many attempts). Stretch a piece of duct tape over the affected area. Press the duct tape onto the skin and gently rub it over the needles to make sure they are stuck. Grasp one end of the tape and quickly rip it off. Repeat with fresh pieces of tape. Adhesive tape and cellophane tape are not very effective. **d.** If a cactus stem or pad is attached, use a plastic comb or two sticks to grasp underneath the stem or pad and flick it away before trying any of the above methods. **2.** Clean and treat the wound with antibiotic ointment and dressing.

Stinging Nettle

The stinging nettle plant has stinging hairs on its stem and leaves. Its effects are not an allergic response but are due to an irritant found in the plant's sap.

What to Look for	What to Do
Immediate onset of intense redness, burning, and itching to the exposed area, lasting for an hour or more	**1.** Wash the area with soap and water. **2.** Apply a cold, wet pack. You could also use colloidal oatmeal, hydrocortisone cream (1%), or calamine lotion. **3.** Give an antihistamine, if desired, following the package directions.

Swallowed (Ingested) Poisonous Plant

What to Look for	What to Do
■ Abdominal pain and cramping ■ Nausea or vomiting ■ Diarrhea ■ Drowsiness ■ Burns, odor, or stains around and inside the mouth	**1.** Rapidly determine: ■ The type of plant, if possible ■ How much was swallowed ■ When it was swallowed **2.** For an alert and awake person, use a mobile phone to call the Poison Control hotline at 1-800-222-1222, even if signs of poisoning are not present. Follow their directions. Most poisonings can be treated through telephone instructions. **3.** For an unresponsive person, check breathing and treat accordingly. Evacuate and seek professional medical care immediately. **4.** Place the person on their left side to delay poison's advance into the intestines and to prevent inhalation of vomit, if vomiting occurs. **5.** **DO NOT** try to induce vomiting or give anything to eat or drink. **6.** Evacuate and seek professional medical care immediately for all mushroom-poisoned people.

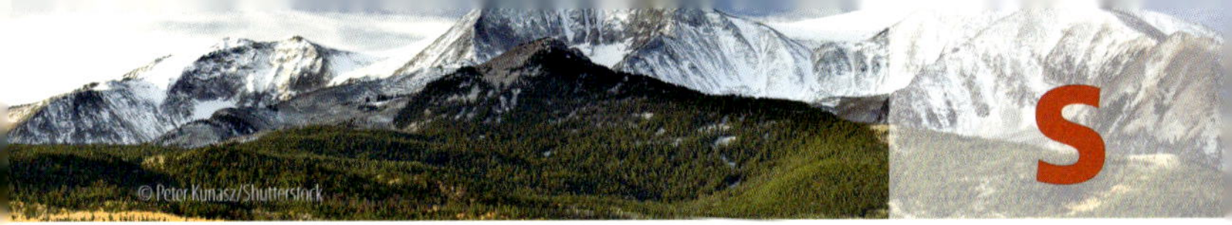

Seizures

Seizures result from a disturbance of the electrical activity in the brain, causing uncontrollable muscle movements. Causes include epilepsy, head injury, brain tumor, stroke, heatstroke, poisoning (including alcohol or drugs), insulin reaction, or high fever.

What to Look for	What to Do
▪ A sudden cry or scream ▪ A sudden loss of responsiveness ▪ Rigid body followed by jerky movement with arching of the back (convulsions) ▪ Foaming at mouth ▪ Drooling from mouth ▪ Grinding of teeth	**1.** Move nearby objects to avoid injury. **2.** Place something soft under the head such as a rolled towel or flat pillow. **DO NOT** use a soft, fluffy pillow. **3.** Time the seizure from start to finish. **4.** Most seizures do not require professional medical care and end in 1 to 2 minutes. Stay with the person until the seizure is over. **5.** Keep bystanders away to protect the person's privacy. **6.** Evacuate for any of the following: ▪ The seizure lasts longer than 5 minutes. ▪ There are a series of seizures, following one after another. ▪ The person has breathing difficulties after the seizure.

Continues

What to Look for	What to Do
■ Blue or gray face and lips ■ Eyes roll upward ■ Loss of bladder or bowel control	■ The person has diabetes or is pregnant. ■ The seizure happened in water. ■ This is the person's first known seizure. ■ The seizure is injury-related. ■ Slow recovery **7.** After the seizure: ■ Keep the airway open by placing the person on their side with their head on a rolled towel. ■ Monitor breathing, and if it stops, give CPR. ■ Allow the person to sleep. ■ Stay with the person until they have fully recovered.

Shock

Shock happens when the body's tissues do not get enough blood. Do not confuse this with an electric shock or "being shocked," as in scared or surprised. Shock is life threatening. Even if there are no signs of shock, you should still follow these procedures for injured people.

What to Look for	What to Do
■ Altered mental status: anxiety and restlessness ■ Pale or ashen, cold, and clammy skin, lips, and nail beds	**1.** Treat injuries. **2.** If responsive, lay the person down. If unresponsive, roll the person onto their side. If a spinal injury is suspected, while rolling the person, keep their nose and navel pointing in the same direction. **3.** Prevent body heat loss by putting blankets/coats under and over the person.

What to Look for	What to Do
▪ Nausea/vomiting ▪ Rapid breathing and heart rate ▪ Unresponsiveness when shock is severe	**4.** If the person does not improve, evacuate and seek professional medical help. **DO NOT** give anything to eat or drink unless medical help is delayed over 1 hour, in which case, sips of water can be given if fluids do not cause nausea and/or vomiting.

Snake and Other Reptile Bites

At least one species of venomous snake is found in every state except Alaska, Hawaii, and Maine **FIGURE 22**. In about 25% of venomous snakebites, there is no venom injected, only fang and tooth wounds (known as a "dry" bite).

For all snake and reptile bites:

- Get the person and bystanders away from the snake or reptile because of the risk of a second bite. A dead snake can still bite even if decapitated.
- Keep the person quiet and still.
- Gently wash the bite with soap and water.

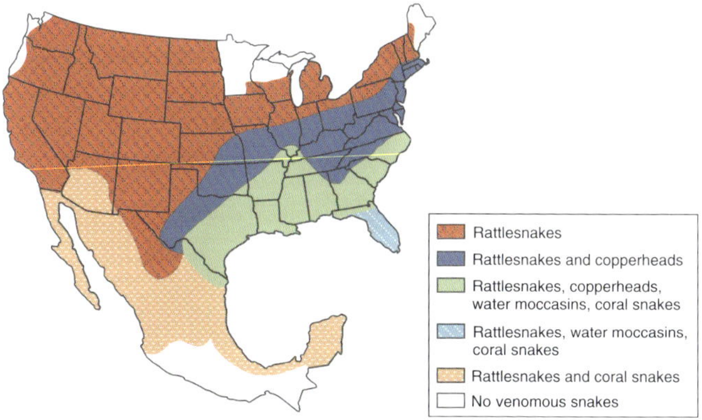

FIGURE 22 Locations of venomous snakes.

Reptile	What to Look for	What to Do
Pit Vipers **FIGURE 23** ■ Rattlesnakes ■ Copperheads ■ Cottonmouths/ Water Moccasins	■ Severe, burning pain at the bite site ■ Two small puncture wounds (person may have only one) ■ Swelling within 10 to 15 minutes; can involve entire extremity	**1.** It is not necessary to capture or kill the snake. **2.** Evacuate and seek professional medical care immediately. When possible, carry the person. If alone and capable, walk slowly.

Reptile	What to Look for	What to Do
Triangular, flat head, wider than the neck; vertical, elliptical pupils (cat's eye); and a heat-sensitive "pit" located between the eye and nostril	▪ Discoloration and blood-filled blisters possible in 6 to 10 hours ▪ Severe cases have nausea, vomiting, sweating, and weakness.	**3.** *Cautions*: **DO NOT** cut the person's skin to drain venom. **DO NOT** use mouth suction. **DO NOT** use any suction device. **DO NOT** apply cold/ice packs. **DO NOT** give alcohol. **DO NOT** apply electrical shock. **DO NOT** use a tourniquet. **DO NOT** apply a pressure bandage.

Coral snakes
Small and very colorful, with a series of bright red, yellow, and black bands going all the way around its body. Every alternate band is yellow, and the snout is black.
It is the most venomous snake in North America, but rarely bites.
	▪ Few immediate signs
	▪ Absence of immediate symptoms is not evidence of a harmless bite.
	▪ Several hours may pass before the onset of:
	  ▪ Nausea
	  ▪ Vomiting
	  ▪ Sweating
	  ▪ Tremors
	  ▪ Drowsiness
	  ▪ Slurred speech
	  ▪ Blurred vision
	  ▪ Swallowing difficulty
	  ▪ Breathing difficulty
		1. Apply mild pressure by wrapping several elastic bandages (eg, Ace) over the bite site and entire extremity.
		2. **DO NOT** cut skin or use suction.
		3. Evacuate and seek professional medical care immediately.

Continues

Reptile	What to Look for	What to Do
Nonvenomous snakes **FIGURE 24** If in doubt, assume the snake is venomous.	■ Leaves a horseshoe shape of tooth marks on skin ■ Possible swelling and tenderness	1. Treat the bite the same as a shallow wound. (Refer to the *Bleeding and Wound Care* section.) 2. Consult with a physician.
Venomous lizards ■ Gila monster (United States and Mexico) ■ Mexican beaded lizard Both lizards may firmly hang on during bite and chew venom into skin	■ Puncture wounds—teeth may break off ■ Swelling and pain, often severe and burning ■ Sweating ■ Vomiting ■ Increased heart rate ■ Shortness of breath	1. Give pain medication. 2. Evacuate. 3. Same as pit vipers.

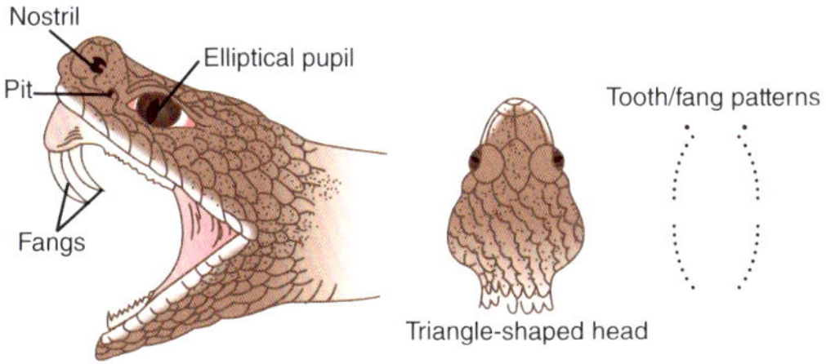

FIGURE 23 Pit viper (venomous snake) characteristics.

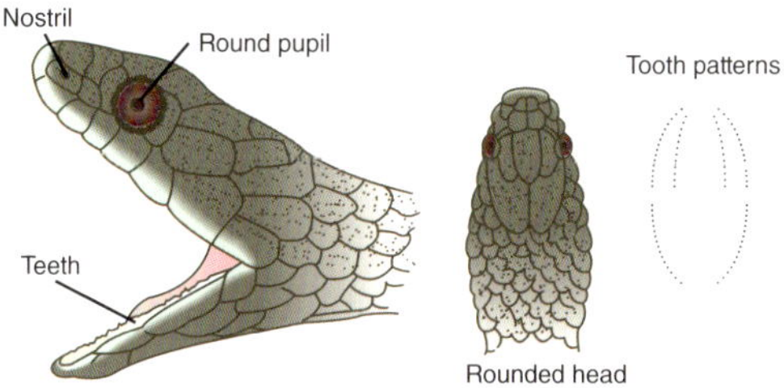

FIGURE 24 Nonvenomous snake characteristics.

Spinal Injury

When a significant cause of injury (eg, a vehicle crash involving ejection, a rollover, or high speeds; a head injury causing unresponsiveness; penetrating wounds of the neck or trunk; or diving into shallow water) occurs, always suspect a spinal injury.

Fully stabilizing a responsive person may not always be necessary, because doing so can be difficult, impractical, impossible, or dangerous to the person.

A *reliable* person does not need to be stabilized in one position if they meet the following criteria:

- Alert, knows name and where they are
- Not intoxicated by drugs/alcohol
- Calm, cooperative
- Lack of painful, distracting injury

An *unreliable* person meets one or more of the following criteria:

- Unresponsive; altered mental status
- Intoxicated by drugs/alcohol
- Combative, confused
- Has a painful, distracting injury

What to Look for	What to Do
In a reliable person: **1.** Reports back pain and leg numbness and tingling **2.** Tenderness/pain when you run fingers all the way down spine (if possible); press each bump of vertebrae and press on depressions produced on each side when you touch or push on the spine bones. **3.** Fails these tests for sensation and movement (test all four extremities): ■ Upper body: **a.** Pinch several fingers while the person has their eyes closed and ask: "Can you feel this? Where am I touching you?" **b.** Ask: "Can you wiggle your fingers?" **c.** Have the person squeeze your hand.	Suspect a spinal injury: **1.** Send for medical help. **DO NOT** attempt to evacuate the person. Wait for trained rescuers with proper equipment. **2.** Leave the person on the ground. Cover to prevent heat loss by log rolling the person, keeping nose and navel pointing in the same direction, and place insulating materials under and over the person. Place padding under the lower back and behind the knees for comfort. **3.** Stabilize the person against movement. Place the person's head between your knees, as this is less tiring than kneeling and holding the person's head with your hands. Improvised cervical collars (eg, SAM Splint, blanket) alone are inadequate. An alternative method that does not require you to hold the person constantly is to improvise "sandbags" by placing dirt, sand, or rocks cushioned with clothing in stuffed sacks or plastic bags and securely placing them on both sides of the person's head.

What to Look for	What to Do
▪ Lower body: **a.** Pinch toes while the person has their eyes closed and ask: "Can you feel this? Where am I touching you?" **b.** Ask: "Can you wiggle your toes?" **c.** Have the person push and pull a foot against your hand.	**4.** Tell the person to remain as still as possible.
If the above are *not* present in a reliable person	Suspect *no* spinal injury. Treat other injuries (eg, wounds, bruises, fractures).
If the person is unreliable and has a significant mechanism of injury (see earlier in this chart for examples)	Assume there is a spinal injury. Use the methods shown earlier in this chart to stabilize the person.

An injured person does not require spinal stabilization if they:

- Are alert, not intoxicated, and have no distracting injuries
- Do not report neck pain or neurological symptoms (eg, tingling, numbness)
- Have no neck tenderness when felt, no loss of sensation when fingers and toes are pinched, and can move their fingers and toes
- Can rotate their neck 45° left and right when requested

Stroke

Stroke is caused by blockage or rupture of a blood vessel in the brain.

A stroke occurs when a brain blood vessel becomes plugged or ruptures so that part of the brain does not get the blood flow it needs.

What to Look for	What to Do
The acronym **F-A-S-T** acts as an assessment tool to help determine if a stroke may have occurred: **F** = Face droops—ask the person to smile. It is abnormal for one side of the face not to move well compared with the other side. **A** = Arm weakness—Ask the person to close their eyes and raise both arms with the palms up for a count of 10 seconds. It is abnormal if one arm drifts downward when held extended. **S** = Speech difficulty—Ask the person to repeat a simple phrase (eg, "The sky is blue."). It is abnormal if the person slurs words, uses the wrong words, or cannot speak at all. **T** = Time to evacuate and seek professional medical care if any of the preceding signs occur. The presence of one of these signs is associated with a high risk of stroke (72%); if all three are present, the risk is as high as 85%.	**1.** Call 9-1-1 immediately. **2.** Monitor responsiveness and breathing. ■ If the person is unresponsive and not breathing, begin CPR. ■ If they are unresponsive and breathing or have fluid or vomit in their mouth, place them on their side in the recovery position. ■ If they are alert, allow them to find a comfortable position with the head and shoulders above the body. **3.** **DO NOT** give the person anything to eat or drink—the throat can be paralyzed, which restricts swallowing and causes choking. **4.** Loosen tight clothing (eg, shirt collars, ties). **5.** Record the time that the stroke may have occurred and give it to medical personnel.

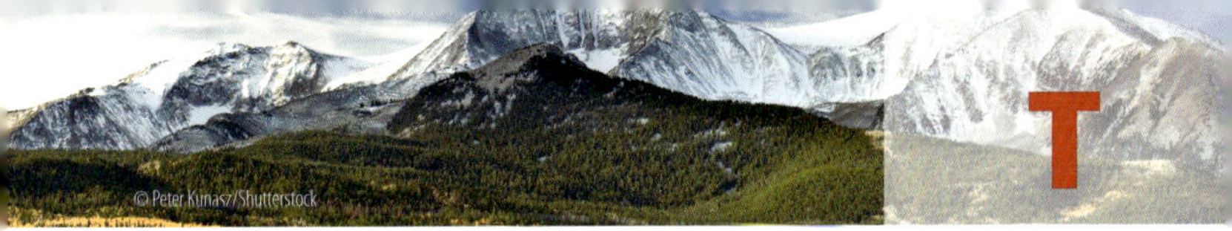

© Peter Kunasz/Shutterstock

Tooth Injuries

Because dental emergencies generally cause considerable pain and anxiety, managing them promptly can provide great relief to the person. Seek dental care for all dental injuries; in most cases, as soon as possible.

What to Look for	What to Do
Object caught between teeth, indicated by: ▪ Person reports that something is caught between their teeth ▪ An object that may or may not be seen (even with a flashlight, it is difficult to see the small object)	**1.** Try to remove the object with dental floss. Guide the floss carefully to avoid cutting the gums. **2.** **DO NOT** try to remove the object with a sharp or pointed instrument. **3.** If unsuccessful, evacuate and seek dental care.

Continues

What to Look for	What to Do
Bitten lip or tongue, indicated by: ▪ Immediate pain ▪ Bleeding ▪ Swelling	**1.** Apply direct pressure to the bleeding area with sterile gauze or a clean cloth. **2.** Clean the area with a cloth. **3.** If swelling is present, apply an ice pack or have the person suck on a popsicle or ice chips. **4.** If the bleeding does not stop, evacuate and seek professional medical care.
Loosened tooth ▪ Apply pressure on either side of each tooth with the fingers to determine looseness. ▪ Any tooth movement, even if it is barely felt, indicates a possibly loose tooth.	**1.** Have the person bite down on a piece of gauze to keep the tooth in place. **DO NOT** remove a partially extracted tooth. **2.** Evacuate and consult a dentist or an oral surgeon immediately.
Toothache, indicated by: ▪ Person reports pain limited to one area of the mouth (although it can be more widespread); pain can also affect the ear, eye, neck, or even the opposite side of the jaw.	**1.** Rinse the person's mouth with warm water. Be sure they don't swallow the water. **2.** Use dental floss to remove any trapped food. **3.** Place an ice pack on the outside of the cheek to reduce swelling. **4.** If available, use a cotton swab to paint the aching tooth with oil of cloves (eugenol) to help suppress the pain. Take care to keep the oil off the gums, lips, and inside surfaces of the cheeks.

What to Look for	What to Do
▪ Person reports a tooth that is sensitive to heat and cold. ▪ Dental decay (identified by tapping the area with a spoon handle or similar object; a diseased tooth will hurt)	**5.** Give over-the-counter (OTC) pain medication (eg, acetaminophen, ibuprofen) according to package directions. **DO NOT** place aspirin on the aching tooth or gum tissues or allow them to dissolve in the mouth. A serious acid burn can result. **6.** Evacuate and seek a dentist.
Broken tooth	**1.** Collect all the tooth or teeth fragments. Depending upon the severity of the injury, a dentist may be able to reattach them. **2.** Rinse the person's mouth with warm water. Be sure they don't swallow the water. **3.** For swelling over the injured area, place an ice pack on the outside of the cheek. **4.** For pain, have the person keep air exposure to a minimum by keeping their mouth closed. Additionally, consider providing OTC pain medication according to package directions, which should be swallowed. **5.** If a jaw fracture is suspected, stabilize the jaw by wrapping a bandage under the chin and over the top of the head. **DO NOT** tie the mouth closed. Be sure to allow enough space for fluids to drain. **6.** Evacuate and seek a dentist immediately. **7.** Transport the fragments as you would a knocked-out tooth (see the next section).

Continues

What to Look for	What to Do
Knocked-out (avulsed) tooth	**1.** Attempt to reimplant the tooth (only if it is a permanent [adult] tooth and the person is unable to see a dentist within 1 hour of the injury): ■ Hold the tooth by the crown (tooth part normally seen when looking into a mouth). **DO NOT** touch the root. ■ If the tooth is dirty, gently rinse it in a bowl of warm water. **DO NOT** scrub or remove any of the attached tissue fragments. ■ Gently push the tooth down into the socket so the top is even with the adjacent teeth. The person can bite down gently on gauze or a handkerchief placed between the teeth. **2.** If unable to reimplant the tooth, control bleeding in the socket (place a dressing in the socket and apply pressure) and keep the knocked-out tooth viable by storing it in a solution (listed in order of preference): ■ Hank's Balanced Salt Solution (Save-A-Tooth) ■ Egg white ■ Coconut water ■ Cow's milk ■ Almond or coconut milk ■ The person's own saliva ■ Wrap in clear plastic wrap **3.** Evacuate and seek a dentist as soon as possible. **4.** *Cautions:* ■ **DO NOT** handle a knocked-out tooth roughly. ■ **DO NOT** touch the root of a knocked-out tooth. ■ **DO NOT** scrub a knocked-out tooth or remove any attached tissue fragments.

What to Look for	What to Do
	▪ **DO NOT** put a knocked-out tooth in water, mouthwash, alcohol, or povidone iodine (Betadine). ▪ **DO NOT** put a knocked-out tooth in reconstituted powdered milk or milk by-products such as yogurt. ▪ **DO NOT** rinse a knocked-out tooth unless you are reinserting it in the socket. ▪ **DO NOT** place a knocked-out tooth in anything that can dry or crush the outside of the tooth.
Infected or abscessed tooth, indicated by: ▪ Swelling of the gums around the affected tooth ▪ Foul breath ▪ Pain that is increased by tapping the tooth on the top with something metal (eg, spoon handle)	**1.** Have the person rinse their mouth several times per day with warm water. Remind them not to swallow the water. **2.** Give OTC pain medication according to package directions. DO NOT have the person suck an aspirin, and DO NOT place an aspirin on the tooth or gum tissue. **3.** An ice pack on the cheek may help. **4.** Use dental floss to remove any trapped food. **5.** Evacuate and seek a dentist.
Cavity—caused by decay or lost filling—indicated by: ▪ Sensitivity to heat, cold, or sweets	**1.** Have the person rinse their mouth with warm water. Be sure they don't swallow the water. **2.** Apply oil of cloves (eugenol) with a cotton swab to the cavity to deaden the pain. DO NOT apply any on the gums or lips, or inside the cheeks.

Continues

What to Look for	What to Do
▪ Sensitivity to touch. (Tap the tooth gently with something metal [eg, spoon handle] on the top and side. This increases the pain in the affected tooth.)	**3.** If available, apply a temporary filling with cavity dental filling paste. Other options include sugarless chewing gum, candle wax, or ski wax. **DO NOT** cover a cavity with cotton if there is any pus discharge or facial swelling. **4.** Evacuate and seek a dentist.
Bleeding from mouth	**1.** Allow blood to drain out of the mouth. **2.** For a bleeding tongue, put a dressing on the wound and apply pressure. **3.** For a cut through a lip, place a rolled dressing between the lip and gum and press another dressing against the outer lip. **4.** Evacuate and seek professional medical care.

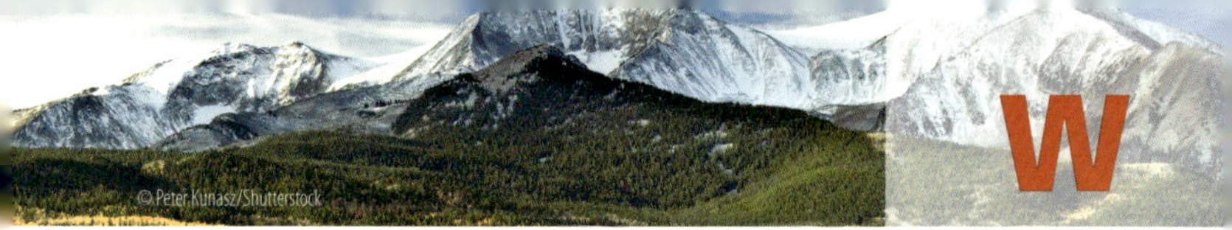

Wild Animal Attacks

Human injuries by wild animals are rare, yet people often fear venturing into wilderness areas. Many of their apprehensions come from myths, ignorance, exaggeration, and sensationalism. Most wild animals try to avoid people, and when attacks do occur, they often result in only minor injuries. Traveling in a group is safer than being alone. In North America, the wild animals that are most commonly reported as interacting with people include bears, bison, moose, cougars, coyotes, and alligators. Not all Injuries are bites. Severe injuries can result from people being thrown in the air, gored by antlers, butted, or trampled on the ground. Injuries include puncture wounds, bites, lacerations, bruises, fractures, rupture of internal organs, and evisceration. The majority of wild animal attacks occur outside of the United States (for "What to Do," see the Bleeding and Wound Care section). Evacuate and seek professional medical care immediately.

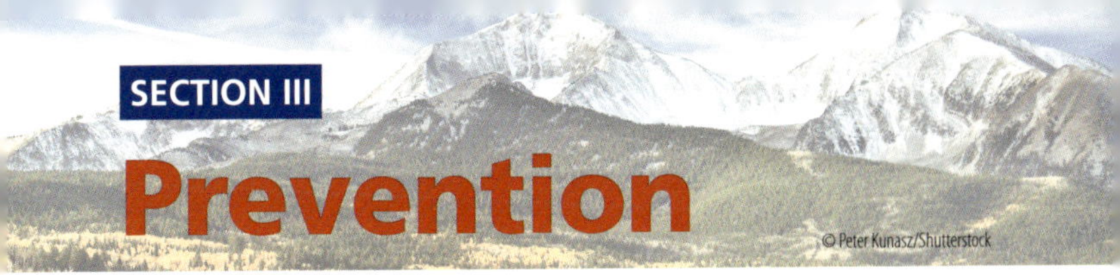

SECTION III

Prevention

© Peter Kunasz/Shutterstock

Signaling for Help

Many emergency conditions require a search for people in distress. Under such circumstances, it is always better if those being sought know how to make their presence and location conspicuous.

Signaling Aircraft

The key to any ground signal is that very few straight lines or right angles exist in nature. Remember that things appear a lot smaller when viewed from the air, and thus, bigger is almost always better. For ground signals, make a large **V** for immediate assistance or an **X** if medical assistance is needed. Make the lines of these signals as large as you can.

Construct your signal using a ratio of six to one (eg, a **V** with sides 12 feet high and 2 feet wide). Contrast is another key to ground signals. Examples of materials to use include toilet paper, strips of plastic tarp, strips of tent material, tree branches, logs, and light-colored rocks. In snow, on the open ground, or on a beach, signals may be tramped or dug into the surface using shadows to make the signals stand out.

Other Signals

A series of three signals in quick succession indicates "help." Examples include three shouts, three shots, three blasts from a whistle, or three flashes from a light.

Use smoke by day and bright flame by night if other signaling devices are not available. Add engine oil, rags soaked in oil, or pieces of rubber to your fire to make black smoke (best against light background). Add green leaves, moss, or a little water to send up billows of white smoke (best against dark background). If tending a fire while waiting for help, keep plenty of fuel at hand. Throw it on the fire the moment an aircraft is heard—it takes time for smoke to form and rise.

A mirror is an effective means of sending a distress signal. On hazy days, aircraft pilots can see the flash of a mirror before survivors can see the aircraft; it is wise to flash the mirror in the direction of a plane when you hear it, even if you cannot see it. Mirror flashes have been spotted by rescue aircraft more than 20 miles (32 km) away.

To use a mirror, follow this procedure:

1. Hold the mirror up to the sun with one hand, and stretch your other hand in front of you, holding up a finger or thumb so it blots out the view of your target.
2. Hit your extended finger or thumb with a reflection of the sun from the mirror.
3. Repeatedly flick the spot of light from the mirror across the finger or thumb and the aircraft.
4. Try to hit the aircraft or rescuers with a flash as much as possible. **DO NOT** attempt to do a series of three flashes—it is too difficult **FIGURE 25**.

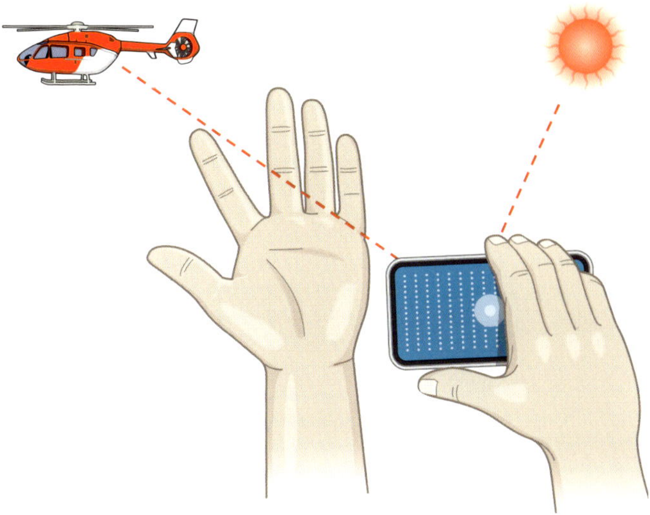

FIGURE 25 Signaling aircraft.

Evacuation

Evacuation refers to moving an injured or ill person to professional medical care. Evacuating a person out of a wilderness area is often difficult, expensive, and time consuming, and it frequently puts rescuers at risk for injury.

Not every cut requires stitches, nor does every burn require professional medical care. It is, however, always best to err on the side of caution. According to the American College of Emergency Physicians, if the answer to any of the following questions is "yes," or if you are unsure, evacuate the person for professional medical care:

- Is the condition life threatening?
- Could the condition worsen if the person is not transported?
- If you do not move the person, will further injury occur?
- Does the person need the medical care of equipment available from outside medical help?
- Would distance, terrain, or weather cause a delay in getting the medical care?
- Is the person unable to travel or participate in the activity (for which they went to a remote location) at a reasonable pace owing to a medical problem?

It is usually best to postpone further travel and initiate evacuation from the wilderness for any person who has the following:

- Worsening symptoms, such as:
  - Altered mental status
  - Unrelieved vomiting or diarrhea
  - An inability to tolerate drinking fluids
  - Losing consciousness for a second time after a head injury
- Debilitating pain
- Inability to travel at a reasonable pace because of a medical problem
- Sustained abdominal pain

- Passage of blood by mouth or rectum (not from an obviously minor source)
- Serious high-altitude illness signs and symptoms
- Infections that worsen despite appropriate treatment
- Chest pain that is not clearly musculoskeletal in origin
- Development of a dysfunctional psychological status that impairs the safety of the person or group
- Large or severe wounds or a wound with complications (eg, open fracture, deformed fracture, a suspected spinal injury, a fracture or dislocation impairing circulation to arm or leg)

Guidelines for Ground Evacuation

If the person is walking out, at least three people should accompany them. If the person is unable to continue, one first aid provider can stay with the person while the others go for help.

If the person is being carried out:

- Send two people to notify authorities that help is needed.
- At least four, preferably six, bearers should carry the stretcher (litter) at all times.
- Over rough terrain, eight carriers (six over smooth trail) should carry the litter 100 yards (91 m) and then rest or rotate with other carriers. It is very physically demanding to carry a loaded litter for more than 15 minutes without a break, especially at high altitude.

Even when rescue help is requested (eg, via mobile phone), a detailed written note describing the situation and person's condition should be completed. When without a mobile or satellite phone, one or two members of the party can carry out a written request for help.

Guidelines for Helicopter Evacuation

Helicopters can reduce the time to professional medical care. Evacuate by helicopter only if the following applies:

- The person's life will be saved.
- The person will have a significantly better chance for full recovery.
- The pilot believes conditions are safe enough for helicopter evacuation.
- Ground evacuation would be dangerous or prolonged, or lacks a sufficient number of rescuers.

Generally, helicopters are not beneficial if ground transport can get the person to the hospital within 30 to 60 minutes or less.

Helicopter Safety Rules

The chief hazards are the main rotor blades and the tail rotor (this appears nearly invisible during operation).

- Always approach the helicopter from the front where the pilot can see you.
- Keep as low as possible when approaching a helicopter.
- Never walk downhill to approach the helicopter. Never walk uphill when exiting a helicopter.
- Approach and board only when the pilot signals it is safe.
- Secure all loose clothing and equipment.
- Never chase an item that has blown away. Wait for the helicopter to land.

- Protect eyes from the rotor downwash.
- If blinded by debris, stop and kneel.
- Someone will come to help.
- **DO NOT** stand in the landing zone.
- Clear debris from the landing zone before the helicopter's arrival.

First Aid Kits

Most injuries and sudden illnesses do not require professional medical care. For all remote locations, it is a good idea to have useful supplies available for emergencies.

A first aid kit's supplies should be customized to include those items that are likely to be used on a regular basis, including nonprescription (over-the-counter) medications. Some medications lose their potency over time, especially after they have been opened; check expiration dates twice per year. Keep all medicines out of the reach of children. Read and follow all directions for proper medication use.

The following list contains useful first-aid kit items. Change the list to meet the needs of situations you are likely to encounter.

Item	Purpose
Micropore paper tape (1- and 2-inch)	Covers blisters and/or blister-prone areas
Elastikon tape (2- and 4-inch)	Covers wounds and blisters
Spenco 2nd Skin (1- and 3-inch)	Covers wounds and blisters

Continues

Item	Purpose
Moleskin/mole foam	Apply over "hot spots" before blister formation. Can be cut in to a "donut shape" to surround blister.
Alcohol hand sanitizer gel (small bottle)	Cleans hands and the area around the wound (not inside wound)
Antibiotic ointment (Polysporin, Neosporin, Bacitracin, triple-antibiotic ointment)	Prevents skin infections that are associated with shallow wounds and makes nonstick dressings
Aloe vera gel (100% gel)	Apply to skin for sunburn or superficial frostbite.
Blister bandage (Blist-O-Ban) (1 package)	Apply over "hot spots" before blister formation.
Irrigation syringe (10 or 20 cc)	Provides pressure irrigation of wounds
Adhesive bandages (various sizes; also known as Band-Aids)	Covers minor wounds
Sterile gauze pads (2 × 2–inch and 4 × 4–inch individually wrapped)	Covers wounds
Nonstick pads	Covers burns, blisters, and scrapes
Self-adhering roller bandage (2 to 4 inches wide; Kerlix, Kling)	Holds dressings in place
Sterile trauma pad (5 × 9–inch, 8 × 10–inch)	Covers large wounds
Elastic roller bandage (4 inches wide; Ace wrap)	Provides compression to reduce the swelling of joint injuries
Adhesive tape—various types available (eg, athletic tape, hypoallergenic tape, waterproof tape)	Secures dressings and splints
Duct tape (very small roll)	Covers skin "hot spots" before blister formation, holds a dressing or splint, and has many other uses

Item	Purpose
Safety pins (2 inches long)	Creates sling from shirttail or sleeve, secures dressings, and drains friction blisters
Triangular bandages	Arm sling, convert into a cravat bandage
Tourniquet	Applies pressure to a limb or extremity in order to limit blood flow during massive bleeding.
Pain and anti-inflammatory medication—for children, use acetaminophen (Tylenol); for adults, use aspirin or ibuprofen (Advil, Motrin)	Treats pain, fever, and swelling. Give only acetaminophen for children. Acetaminophen does not reduce swelling.
Decongestant tablets (eg, Sudafed) Decongestant spray (eg, Afrin, Neo-Synephrine)	Relieves nasal and upper respiratory congestion of viral colds, allergies, and sinus infections. Spray can be helpful in controlling nosebleeds.
Antihistamine (eg, Benadryl)	Relieves allergy symptoms and treats poison ivy or oak itching and rash. It reduces nausea and motion sickness, causes drowsiness, and induces sleep.
Hydrocortisone cream, 1%	Soothes inflammation associated with insect bites and stings, poison ivy and oak, and other allergic skin rashes. It may be too weak for some conditions.
Commercial sports drink packets (eg, Gatorade)	Treats heat stress, dehydration, and "water intoxication" when too much water has been consumed and sodium has been depleted from body
Sunscreen lotion (with at least SPF 15)	Prevents sunburn and windburn

Continues

Item	Purpose
Lip balm (with at least SPF 15)	Prevents sunburn and chapping of lips and soothes cold sores
Insect repellent with DEET (diethyltoluamide, <30%)	Repels insects. For children, use no more than 10% DEET. Permethrin on clothes repels ticks.
Antacids tablets (eg, Tums and Rolaids)	Treats heartburn and acid indigestion
Antidiarrheal tablets (eg, Pepto-Bismol and Imodium A-D)	Treats diarrhea
Anticonstipation tablets (eg, Metamucil)	Treats constipation
Scissors—various types available	Cut dressings, bandages, and clothing
Tweezers (angled tip)	Removes splinters and ticks
Thermometer, digital (75° F to 105° F)	Measures fever
SAM splint	Stabilizes broken bones and dislocations
Medical exam gloves (eg, disposable nitrile gloves)	Protects against potentially infected blood and body fluids
Mouth-to-barrier device	Protects against potential infection during CPR
Emergency blanket (eg, state highway department trash bags; household polyethylene trash bags; "space blanket" made of Mylar, although may tear in wind)	Protects against body heat loss and weather (wind, rain, and snow)
Small notebook/pencil	Records information
Small first aid manual	Quick reference during an emergency and is used for learning and reviewing first aid procedures

Basic Survival Kit: The Bare Essentials

Carry at least the items in this kit whenever you are in remote areas.

Minimal Items	Purpose
One or two large, heavy-duty plastic bags (similar to state highway department trash bags), household polyethylene trash bags, or emergency blanket ("space blanket") made of Mylar, although it may tear in wind	Protects against weather (wind, rain, snow). Wear one trash bag by cutting hole in bottom of bag for head to fit through; use the second bag to cover legs.
Whistle*	Signal for help.
Signal mirror**	Signal for help.
Metal match with striker (magnesium)	Start a fire.
Waterproof match case containing windproof/ waterproof matches	Start a fire.
Waterproof match case or empty film canister containing several cotton balls smeared with petroleum jelly (Vaseline)	Petroleum jelly is flammable. Make tinder using cotton balls smeared with petroleum jelly. When using, open the cotton ball to catch sparks from metal match.
Knife (multitool) and/or wire blade survival saw	Used for cutting

Continues

Minimal Items	Purpose
Food***	Provides calories and a psychological boost

* Whistle: A whistle is far superior to shouting. The whistle will carry for 0.5 to 2.0 miles or more in the wilderness, whereas your voice may only carry a few hundred yards. You will be able to signal for longer periods of time. Give three blasts in succession, repeated at intervals, to get attention. New high-tech whistles such as the "Storm" (from All-Weather Safety Whistle Co.) and the "Fox 40" (from Fox 40 International) and the smaller, more compact versions of these super whistles, the Windstorm and the Fox 40 Mini CMG, are much louder than police or referee whistles.

** Signal mirror: A mirror of 4 × 5 inches (standard US Coast Guard size) or 3 × 5 inches is ideal, but the smaller 2 × 3–inch size also works well. Specially made glass and plastic signal mirrors are available. If you do not have a mirror, improvise using any piece of metal (polish it with fine sand or dirt), foil, or any shiny object. A mirror works even on overcast days and with moonlight, although with reduced range.

*** Food: Good items to carry include energy bars, candy bars, hard candy (eg, lemon drops), powdered chocolate, dehydrated soup, or MREs (meals ready to eat). Discard any with soon-to-lapse expiration dates.

Prevention: Altitude Illness

1. **DO NOT** rush to your destination. At higher elevations, start slowly and avoid overexertion. Those not accustomed to high altitudes should not ascend rapidly to sleeping altitudes greater than 10,000 feet and should spend 2 to 3 nights at 8,000 to 10,000 feet before going higher, with 1 extra night for every 2,000 to 3,000 feet. You can climb or ski higher during the day and return to a lower elevation at night ("climb or ski high, sleep low").

2. Drink lots of water (see the *Prevention: Dehydration* section for information).
3. Eat a high-carbohydrate diet because the appetite is often suppressed; also, food may be less available, and energy needs are greater.
4. **DO NOT** take sleeping pills because they cause shallow breathing while sleeping.
5. **DO NOT** smoke because it increases carbon monoxide blood levels, lessening the body's ability to use oxygen.
6. Ask your physician about the possible use of the medication acetazolamide (Diamox), which can prevent symptoms of acute mountain illness.

Prevention: Avalanche Burial

An avalanche is a mass of snow that slides down a mountainside.

1. Before going into potential avalanche country, call the nearest avalanche hotline to get the latest information about mountain weather, snow, and avalanche conditions.
2. Only one person at a time should go onto a slope that looks risky. Other people should serve as spotters from a safe location.
3. Avoid the center of open slopes. Cross an open slope at the very top or bottom.
4. Stay on shallow slopes. Avalanches most often start on slopes that are 30° to 45°. Areas where avalanches occur year after year should be avoided **FIGURE 26**.
5. **DO NOT** travel alone.

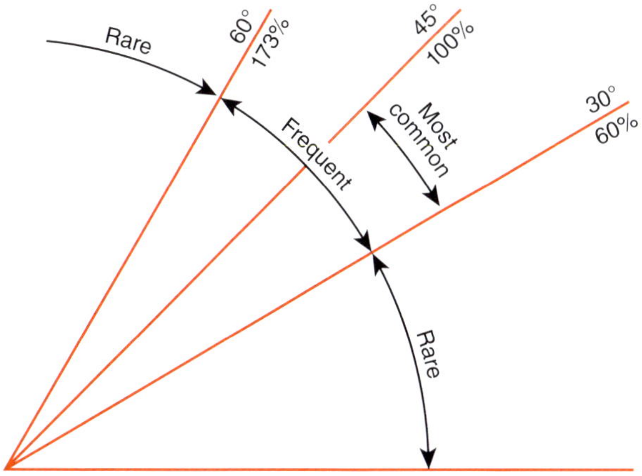

FIGURE 26 Avalanche slope angles.

6. If caught in an avalanche:
- Try to escape to the side of the avalanche. **DO NOT** try to outrun by going downhill on skis or snowmobile.
- Try to grab a tree.
- Try to swim with the moving snow, similar to body surfing in the ocean.
- Try to get away from a snowmobile, and get rid of ski poles.
- Try to burst through the surface before the avalanche stops and clear a breathing space over your mouth.

Prevention: Bear Attack

Bear attacks rarely happen. Most encounters end without injury.

1. Avoid areas where high bear activity has been recently reported.
2. Try to avoid surprising a bear by making noise; hike with a group.
3. Hike during daylight hours.
4. Recognize the signs of a bear (eg, footprints, droppings, and scratches against trees with hair left).
5. Avoid using highly odorous foods that may attract a bear.
6. Properly store your food and garbage at all times except when they are being transported, prepared, or used. Store all food in vehicles or high in a tree—away from the sleeping area. Deposit garbage in a refuse container or store as you would food. **DO NOT** bury it.
7. Never feed bears; never approach bears.
8. If a bear charges you:
   - **DO NOT** run—you cannot outrun a bear; try to remain calm.
   - **DO NOT** climb a tree—black bears and young grizzlies can climb trees.
   - **DO NOT** make quick movements; talk to the bear in a normal, monotone voice.
   - **DO NOT** stare directly at the bear.
   - If you have pepper spray, prepare to use it.

- If the bear makes a bluff charge, stand quietly in a nonaggressive stance. In most cases, the bear stops the charge without making contact or causing injury. At this point, leave the area in the opposite direction from the bear.
- For a black bear without cubs, try to chase it off with mild aggression: yell, shout, blow a whistle, throw rocks, and bang pots. If the bear does not leave, back away and leave the area.

9. During an attack:

- Keep a backpack on for protection.
- If you have pepper spray (oil-based capsaicin), spray the bear's eyes when the bear gets within about 20 feet. Continue spraying until the bear stops its charge; the spray lasts from 4 to 9 seconds.
- If it is a black bear, fight back by yelling, throwing rocks or sticks or whatever is available, and hitting and gouging the bear with your feet, fists, sticks, rocks, shovels—anything you have **FIGURE 27**.
- If it is a brown bear (grizzly, Kodiak), play dead. Drop to the ground as the bear touches you, not before, and curl into a ball, covering your neck and head with your hands and arms. **DO NOT** struggle or fight back, and keep quiet. If the bear swats at you, roll with it. Stay facedown and **DO NOT** look around, and **DO NOT** get up until you are sure it is gone.

If any bear preys on you, try to get away, shout for help, fight for your life, and defend yourself with anything available.

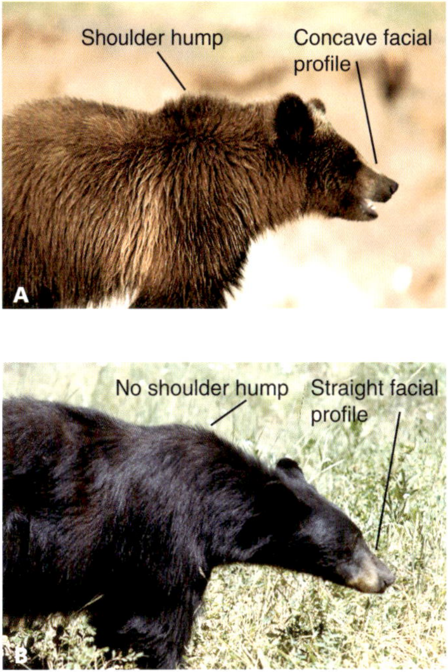

FIGURE 27 A. Brown (grizzly) bear. **B.** Black bear.
Courtesy of John Good/Yellowstone National Park.

Prevention: Blisters

1. Buy shoes or boots with adequate room in the toe box and with a good fit in the heel. They should be a size to a size and a half larger than your dress shoes.
2. Wear socks made of a moisture-wicking fabric (CoolMax) or polypropylene next to the foot to wick moisture away from the foot. Corn starch, talcum powder, baby powder, and antiperspirant also help to keep feet dry.
3. Wear a second pair of socks to prevent friction on the foot itself. Do not wear cotton socks.
4. Coat areas of the feet prone to blister with a blister–chafing prevention agent such as petroleum jelly or A & D (per company website) ointment, or apply micropore paper tape.
5. Stop whenever you feel a hot spot developing, and cover the area with micropore paper tape, Spenco 2nd Skin, moleskin, or Elastikon.
6. Change wet socks into dry ones when possible.

Prevention: Cold-Related Emergencies

If venturing into the wilderness in cold weather, you should have, at a minimum, a wire saw, fire starter, and a Mylar emergency blanket.

Temperature (°F)

Wind (mph)	40	35	30	25	20	15	10	5	0	−5	−10	−15	−20	−25	−30	−35	−40	−45
Calm	40	35	30	25	20	15	10	5	0	−5	−10	−15	−20	−25	−30	−35	−40	−45
5	36	31	25	19	13	7	1	−5	−11	−16	−22	−28	−34	−40	−46	−52	−57	−63
10	34	27	21	15	9	−4	−4	−10	−16	−22	−28	−35	−41	−47	−53	−59	−66	−72
15	32	25	19	13	6	−7	−7	−13	−19	−26	−32	−39	−45	−51	−58	−64	−71	−77
20	30	24	17	11	4	−9	−9	−15	−22	−29	−35	−42	−48	−55	−61	−68	−74	−81
25	29	23	16	9	3	−11	−11	−17	−24	−31	−37	−44	−51	−58	−64	−71	−78	−84
30	28	22	15	8	1	−12	−12	−19	−26	−33	−39	−46	−53	−60	−67	−73	−80	−87
35	28	21	14	7	0	−14	−14	−21	−27	−34	−41	−48	−55	−62	−69	−76	−82	−89
40	27	20	13	6	−1	−8	−15	−22	−29	−36	−43	−50	−57	−64	−71	−78	−84	−91
45	26	19	12	5	−2	−9	−16	−23	−30	−37	−44	−51	−58	−65	−72	−79	−86	−93
50	26	19	12	4	−3	−10	−17	−24	−31	−38	−45	−52	−60	−67	−74	−81	−88	−95
55	25	18	11	4	−3	−11	−18	−25	−32	−39	−46	−54	−61	−68	−75	−82	−89	−97
60	25	17	10	3	−4	−11	−19	−26	−33	−33	−33	−33	−33	−33	−76	−84	−91	−98

Frostbite Times: 30 minutes, 10 minutes, 5 minutes

Wind Chill (°F) = $35.74 + 0.6215T - 35.75(V^{0.16}) + 0.4275T(V^{0.16})$

Where, T=Air Temperature (°F) V=Wind Speed (mph)

FIGURE 28 Windchill Chart.

Courtesy of National Weather Service/NOAA.

Seek and create shelter from cold, wind, snow, and rain:

1. If possible, retreat to timbered areas for shelter construction and fire.
2. Use natural shelters: the windless side of ridges, rock croppings, slope depressions, snow blocks, a snow hole at the base of standing trees, dense stands of trees, or downed trees.
3. Improvise a windbreak or shelter from stacked rocks or snow blocks, tree trunks, limbs, and bark slabs and evergreen boughs, or dig a snow cave or snow trench with a cover **FIGURE 28**.

Conserve, Share, and Create Warmth

1. Conserve body heat by putting on extra clothing. Replace damp clothing and socks. Loosen boot laces to increase circulation. Use a sleeping pad (Ensolite) or evergreen boughs to insulate the body from the ground. Place hands in your armpits or crotch.
2. Share body heat. Sit or lie front to back or back to back. Warm the hands and feet of the injured person or companion.
3. Create body heat. Nibble high-energy goods: candy, nuts, or granola bar. Sip water that is kept warm with body heat. Use a solid fuel hand warmer, igniting both ends of fuel stick (good for 4 hours of heat). Do isometric exercises (exercises done in one position, such as hand press; sit up with back straight and arms straight out in front, then grasp hands together and press firmly) to stir the body's circulation system.
4. Build a fire. Find dry wood: dead lower branches and bark from underside of trees. Look under downed trees and inside of dead logs for dry kindling. Wet wood will burn as it dries in a strong fire. Select a sheltered area, protected from strong winds, as the site for an emergency campfire. Under snow conditions, build a fire base first, with 4-inch diameter or larger pieces of wood (use wire saw). Put fire starter on the base. Surround the fire starter with branches to hold kindling above the fire starter, and then place a hatch work of kindling and slightly larger wood on the branches. Light the fire starter, and blow lightly to help its flame ignite kindling. Add progressively larger wood to the flame area.

5. **DO NOT** drink alcoholic beverages because they:
   - Cause frequent urination, resulting in dehydration
   - Dilate the skin's blood vessels, allowing more heat loss
6. Prevent heat loss. Remember that the body loses heat by respiration, evaporation, conduction, radiation, and convection.
   - To prevent loss by respiration, cover the mouth and nose with loosely woven wool or fleece.
   - To reduce evaporation through excessive perspiration, wear layers of clothing that allow your skin to breathe.
   - To avoid loss by conduction, use a sleeping pad (Ensolite) and/or other cover between the body and a cold, wet surface. This insulation is particularly important if you are already wet.
   - To prevent loss by radiation, keep the head, hands, and feet covered.
   - To prevent loss by convection, protect the body from the wind. A Mylar emergency blanket is a very effective wind block and is also waterproof.

Clothing

1. Wear a base or first layer of clothing made of polypropylene.
2. Wear an insulating or second layer consisting of shirt and pants made of wool, fleece, or down.
3. Wear outer layers made of a windproof and water-resistant jacket that is worn loosely.

4. **DO NOT** wear cotton, as it does not wick sweat and will cool you rapidly if it gets wet.
5. Wear a stocking cap to insulate the head and retain heat. It should be large enough to cover the ears.
6. Wear a thin pair of gloves (or liners) inside a heavy wool or fleece mitten inside a Gore-Tex shell.
7. Remove layers as you warm up to prevent excessive sweating.
8. Keep clothing dry from rain, snow, and sweat.
9. **DO NOT** wear shoes or boots that are too small, or tie them so tightly that they restrict blood flow. **DO NOT** wear too many socks.

Prevention: Dehydration

The body operates more efficiently when it is well hydrated. Dehydration can increase the severity of most of the conditions described in this field guide, making them more difficult to deal with.

How Much Fluid to Drink?

The Institute of Medicine recommends 13 8-oz. cups of water and other beverages for men; for women, about 9 cups.

Pay special attention to fluid intake when:

- You are physically active.
- The air temperature exceeds 80°F.
- There is low humidity.
- You are at elevations above 5,000 feet.

How can you tell whether you are drinking enough?

- Check your urine—scanty, strong-smelling, dark urine signals that you need to drink more.
- Remember that the color of urine can be affected by medications, vitamins, and diet.
- If you feel thirsty, you are already about 1% to 2% dehydrated.

Can you drink too much water?

- If you overhydrate (drink too much), sodium concentrations can drop (hyponatremia), allowing water to leak into brain cells, causing headache, confusion, personality changes, and even seizures, coma, or death.
- During physical activity, stay within the range of about 1.5 to 3 cups per hour.

Can commercial sports drinks be used?

- During strenuous physical activity in hot environments lasting over 1 hour, commercial sport drinks may be used.
- **DO NOT** take salt tablets.
- Snack foods can be useful if they contain some sodium.

Prevention: Drowning (Submersion/Immersion)

1. Acquire swimming, rescue, and lifesaving skills.
2. Learn how to row a boat and paddle a raft and canoe safely.
3. Children should be supervised by an adult when they are near or in the water.

4. Everyone on a boat, canoe, or raft should wear a US Coast Guard–approved personal flotation device that will support the person with the head above water, even if the person is unresponsive.

Prevention: Heat Stress

1. Keep as cool as possible.
   - Avoid direct sunlight when possible.
   - Wipe cool water on exposed areas of the skin and/or place wet towels or ice bags on the body and/or dampen clothing.
   - Take cool baths or showers.
   - Dip clothing into water periodically, if possible.
2. Wear lightweight, porous, loose-fitting clothing that reflects heat, facilitates evaporative heat loss, and allows air to circulate around your body.
3. Wear a broad-brimmed hat.
4. Apply sunscreen with minimum SPF 15.
5. Avoid, when possible, strenuous physical activity, particularly in the sun and during the hottest part of the day **FIGURE 29**.
6. Drink enough water. Drink 1 cup (8 oz.) every half-hour during strenuous activity. (See *Prevention: Dehydration* section.)
7. **DO NOT** use salt tablets.
8. **DO NOT** drink alcoholic beverages (eg, beer and wine).
9. Rest frequently in shade.
10. Adapt to the heat (acclimate) by exercising in the heat 60 to 90 minutes each day for 1 to 2 weeks.

Temperature (°F)

Relative Humidity (%)	80	82	84	86	88	90	92	94	96	98	100	102	104	106	108	110
40	80	81	83	85	88	91	94	97	101	105	109	114	119	124	130	136
45	80	82	84	87	89	93	96	100	104	109	114	119	124	130	137	
50	81	83	85	88	91	95	99	103	108	113	118	124	131	137		
55	81	84	86	89	93	97	101	106	112	117	124	130	137			
60	82	84	88	91	95	100	105	110	116	123	129	137				
65	82	85	89	93	98	103	108	114	121	128	136					
70	83	86	90	95	100	105	112	119	126	134						
75	84	88	92	97	103	109	116	124	132							
80	84	89	94	100	106	113	121	129								
85	85	90	96	102	110	117	126	135								
90	86	91	98	105	113	122	131									
95	86	93	100	108	117	127										
100	87	95	103	112	121	132										

Likelihood of Heat Disorders with Prolonged Exposure or Strenuous Activity

Caution | Extreme caution | Danger | Extreme danger

FIGURE 29 Heat index.

Courtesy of NOAA.

Prevention: Insect Stings (Bees, Wasps, Hornets, and Yellow Jackets)

1. **DO NOT** walk barefoot.
2. Insect repellents do not work against stinging insects.

3. **DO NOT** swat or flail at a flying insect. If need be, gently brush it aside or patiently wait for it to leave.
4. **DO NOT** drink from open beverage cans. Attracted by the sweet beverage, stinging insects will crawl inside a can.
5. When eating outdoors, try to keep food covered at all times.
6. **DO NOT** wear sweet-smelling fragrances, such as perfumes, hair sprays, colognes, or deodorants.
7. **DO NOT** wear bright-colored clothing with flowery patterns, which attracts flying insects.
8. Wear long pants and long-sleeved shirts.

Prevention: Lightning Strike

If you can see lightning and/or hear thunder, you are already in danger. Louder or more frequent thunder indicates that lightning activity is approaching, increasing the risk for lightning injury or death. Estimate the distance in miles you are from a lightning flash by counting in seconds the time from when the flash is seen until the time the thunder is heard, and divide that number by five.

Use the "30-30 rule"—when the time between seeing the flash (lightning) and hearing the bang (thunder) is less than 30 seconds (this is the first "30"), meaning the lightning is less than 6 miles away, you should be in or seek a safer location. Outdoor activities should not be resumed until at least 30 minutes (second "30") after the last lighting is seen or thunder heard.

1. When outdoors during a lightning/thunderstorm:
   - Avoid water (lakes, rivers, pools, etc).
   - Avoid high ground.
   - Avoid open spaces where you are one of the tallest objects.
   - Avoid a single tree or other high object (eg, rock and bush).
   - Avoid all metal objects including fences, machinery, etc.
   - Avoid small, isolated sheds, rain shelters, etc.

When possible, find shelter in a substantial building or in a fully enclosed metal vehicle such as a car or truck with the windows completely shut. **DO NOT** touch any of the vehicle's interior metal.

2. If lightning is striking nearby when you are outside:
   - Squat like a baseball catcher. Put your feet together. Place your hands over your ears to minimize hearing damage from thunder. **DO NOT** lie flat on the ground because the current from a lightning strike can spread widely.
   - A group of people should spread out and stay a minimum of 15 feet apart.
3. If caught outdoors and no shelter is nearby:
   - Find a low spot away from trees, fences, and poles.
   - If you are in a forest, take shelter under the shorter trees or low brush.
   - If you feel your skin tingle or hair stand on end, squat down like baseball catcher.
4. If boating, try to get to shore as soon as possible.

5. When indoors:
   - Stay away from fireplaces, metal pipes, and open doors and windows.
   - **DO NOT** use a plugged-in telephone (mobile phones are safe).
   - Turn off, unplug, and stay away from appliances, power tools, TV sets, etc.

Prevention: Mosquito Bites

1. Wear protective clothing during dawn and dusk or in areas where mosquitoes are active: long pants, long-sleeved shirt, and socks and shoes. For some areas, consider mosquito netting draped over a hat to protect face and neck.
2. Apply insect repellent containing DEET on exposed skin. **DO NOT** use a product with more than 30% DEET. **DO NOT** exceed 10% DEET for children younger than 5 years of age.
3. Apply permethrin only on clothing, not on the skin (permethrin kills insects; it is not a repellant).
4. Limit outdoor activities or take precautions given the above at dawn and dusk.

Prevention: Mountain Lion Attack

1. Travel with others.
2. Keep small children close.
3. Obey warning signs or notices of mountain lion activity.
4. If you encounter a mountain lion:

- **DO NOT** approach it; slowly back away. **DO NOT** turn your back to it.
- **DO NOT** run: it may trigger an attack.
- **DO NOT** make direct eye contact.
- Appear larger than you are: raise arms above your head and make steady waving motions.
- Yell or shout.
- If small children are with you, pick them up.
- If attacked, use anything as a weapon: a rock, branch, knife, or other hard object. If you have it, use pepper spray (oil-based capsaicin).

Prevention: Poisonous Plant Dermatitis

1. Learn to recognize and avoid poison ivy, poison oak, and poison sumac.
2. Wear long pants and long-sleeve shirts as protective clothing.
3. Apply an appropriate over-the-counter barrier cream (eg, Ivy Block, Work Shield). Replenish the barrier protection every 4 to 6 hours when possible.
4. Wash or dispose of all contaminated clothing.

Prevention: Snakebite

1. **DO NOT** handle venomous snakes; keep away but do not kill them.

2. **DO NOT** hike and camp in snake-infested areas; avoid caves, rock crevices, dens, stonewalls, and wood piles.
3. Watch where you sit and step; **DO NOT** sit on or step over logs until closely checked. **DO NOT** reach into holes or hidden ledges.
4. Wear protective gear such as boots, long pants, and long-sleeved shirts.
5. **DO NOT** handle a dead venomous snake. The reflex action of the jaws can still inflict a bite 20 minutes or more after the snake is dead, even if decapitated.
6. **DO NOT** surprise or corner a snake. Use a walking stick to prod uncleared ground, and make noise so a snake can sense you coming.
7. Check bedding, clothing, and shoes/boots before use.

Prevention: Tick Bite

Ticks like to rest on low-lying brush and "catch a ride" on a passing animal or person. Areas with a high risk of ticks are wooded areas, low-growing grassland, and the seashore.

Ways to reduce chances of getting a tick bite include the following:

1. Avoid tick-infested areas, when possible.
2. In tick-infested areas, stay in the center of paths, avoid sitting on the ground, and check clothing.
3. Dress properly.

- Wear light-colored clothing so ticks can be seen more easily and removed before becoming attached.
- Wear a long-sleeved shirt that fits tightly at the wrists and neck, and tuck your shirt into your pants.
- Wear long pants; tuck pant legs into boots or socks, or use masking or duct tape to secure pant legs tightly to socks, shoes, or boots.

4. After coming indoors, shower or bathe. Look and feel your entire body for ticks, especially in areas that have hair or where clothing was tight. Have a companion or use a mirror to check the scalp, behind and in the ears, neck, back, and behind the knees.
5. Use chemicals:
   - Apply insect repellents containing EPA-approved DEET to clothes and exposed skin. Avoid high-concentration products (more than 30% DEET) on the skin. **DO NOT** inhale or ingest DEET-containing products or get them in your eyes. **DO NOT** use products with more than 10% DEET on children under 5 years.
   - Apply 0.5% permethrin (kills ticks on contact) only to clothing and not the skin. Apply according to label instructions. Applications to shoes, socks, cuffs, and pant legs are most effective against ticks.

Prevention: Waterborne Diseases

There are three main ways of making water safe to drink: boiling, chemicals, and special filters. Before using any of these methods, cloudy or dirty water should first be filtered through a clean cloth or through an appropriate commercial filter.

Boiling

Bringing water to a full boil for 1 full minute at any altitude makes the water safe to drink.

Chemicals

Both iodine and chlorine are inexpensive and are available in tablet or liquid form. Iodine is preferred but should *not* be used if these conditions exist:

- Thyroid disease
- Iodine allergy
- Pregnancy

In all other people, it should not be used for more than a few months.

Iodine does not kill *Cryptosporidium*. Chemicals take longer to work in cold water and require larger amounts for cloudy or dirty water. Follow the manufacturer's directions concerning the amount administered.

Special Filters

Filters are expensive but simple to use. Filters are *not* a reliable method of removing viruses. (LifeStraw Personal Portable Water Filter is an example of a water filter that eliminates bacteria.)

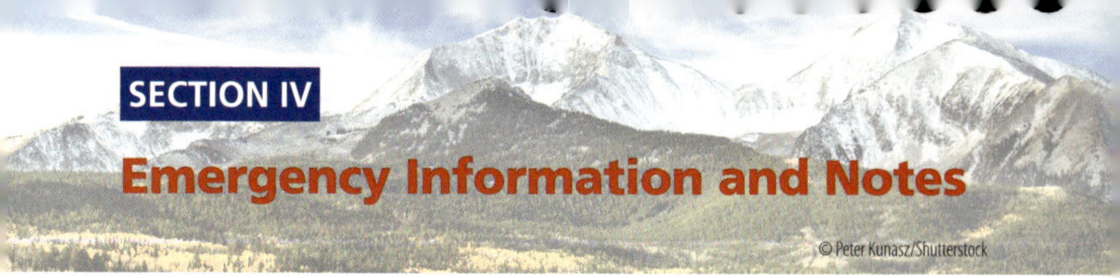

SECTION IV

Emergency Information and Notes

© Peter Kunasz/Shutterstock

Emergency Telephone Numbers and Information

Local Emergency Number **(Usually 9-1-1)**: ....

On-site Emergency Response Number: ....

Poison Control Center: **1-800-222-1222**

National Suicide Prevention Lifeline: **9-8-8**

Physician's Name and Number: ....

Neighbor's Name and Number: ....

Relative's Name and Number: ....

Your Home/Residence

Address: ....

Telephone Number: ....

Nearest Intersection or Landmark: ....

Notes:

Notes:

Notes:

Notes: